# THE COMPASSIONATE MIND APPROACH
# TO BEATING OVEREATING
## USING COMPASSION FOCUSED THERAPY

### KEN GOSS

ROBINSON

Constable London
Constable & Robinson Ltd
3 The Lanchesters
162 Fulham Palace Road
London W6 9ER
www.constablerobinson.com

First published in the UK by Robinson,
an imprint of Constable & Robinson Ltd, 2011

**Important Note**
This book is not intended as a substitute for medical advice or treatment.
Any person with a condition requiring medical attention should consult a
qualified medical practitioner or suitable therapist.

ISBN: 978-1-84529-877-7

Typeset by TW Typesetting, Plymouth, Devon

Printed and bound in the EU

1 3 5 7 9 10 8 6 4 2

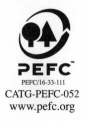

PEFC
PEFC/16-33-111
CATG-PEFC-052
www.pefc.org

# Contents

Introduction by Paul Gilbert ix

Acknowledgements xiii

How to use this book xv

**1 Understanding our relationship with food**

What does a 'compassionate mind' approach mean? 1

Understanding the problem: why we love to eat 2

The perils of modern societies and supermarkets 7

Our need for compassion 9

Moving away from moral judgements about eating 10

How this books works 13

**2 Making sense of overeating, part 1: how our bodies work**

When survival skills backfire 19

Body issues 20

Health issues 23

Food, eating and the need for self-compassion 27

What is a 'healthy body weight'? 29

How our bodies regulate their own weight: the 'set-point system' 31

Overeating, the set point and the hunger–satiety system 32

What we take into our bodies 33

Our pattern of eating 37

The energy we use 45

Summary 48

3 **Making sense of overeating, part 2: eating and our feelings**

Learning to eat 51

Understanding our emotions 53

How are food and emotions linked? 58

Overeating, rules and self-criticism 63

Summary 67

4 **The compassionate mind**

What is compassion and why is it important? 68

Different states of mind 70

Food and our states of mind 73

Shifting towards a compassionate mind 82

Our compassionate mind: an overview 83

Our compassionate mind: the bigger picture 85

Summary 92

5 **Preparing your mind for compassion**

Working with imagery 94

Choosing what we pay attention to 95

*Exercise 5.1: Mindful attention* 98

Activating your soothing system 99

*Exercise 5.2: Soothing breathing rhythm* 100

*Exercise 5.3: Imagining your safe place* 103

Switching on the compassionate mind 105

Exercises to develop the compassionate mind 107

*Exercise 5.4: Envisaging the compassionate self* 110

*Exercise 5.5: You at your best* 112

*Exercise 5.6: Focusing compassion on others* 115

*Exercise 5.7: Compassion flowing out to others in difficulty*   115

*Exercise 5.8: Compassion for people who overeat*   117

*Exercise 5.9: Compassion flowing into you: using your memories*   119

*Exercise 5.10: Creating a compassionate companion*   121

*Exercise 5.11: Using your compassionate companion to help you*   126

*Exercise 5.12: Being the focus of self-compassion*   127

*Exercise 5.13: Focusing self-compassion on a specific problem*   128

Summary   129

**6   Developing the skills of self-compassion**

Managing distress compassionately   131

Learning to activate our affiliative soothing/contentment system   132

*Exercise 6.1: Learning to tolerate distress*   142

Compassionate thinking and behaviour   144

*Exercise 6.2: Compassionate thought balancing*   144

*Exercise 6.3: Getting outside your mindset*   146

Keeping diaries of your practice   152

Blocks to compassion   152

*Exercise 6.4: My personal blocks to experiencing compassion from others*   159

*Exercise 6.5: My personal blocks to developing self-compassion*   159

*Exercise 6.6: Coping with blocks to compassion from others*   160

*Exercise 6.7: Coping with blocks to self-compassion*   160

Summary   161

**7   Why do we overeat? A compassionate mind approach**

What a compassionate 'formulation' for overeating involves   164

Eating as a safety strategy   166

Exploring Alison's compassionate formulation for overeating   168

Why draw up a compassionate formulation for overeating?    174

Making your own compassionate formulation    175

    *Exercise 7.1: Talking to your compassionate image*    176

    *Exercise 7.2: Writing a compassionate life story*    177

    *Exercise 7.3: Using a compassionate formulation form*    177

Summary    183

**8   Understanding your current eating pattern**

Using an eating diary    184

Blocks to monitoring    189

Using your diary to make sense of your eating    195

Making sense of Alison's diary    199

Summary    203

**9   How does your overeating work now?**

Overeating and the 'three systems' of emotional regulation    204

How overeating may help us manage emotions    206

Putting it all together: a new compassionate formulation for your overeating    212

    *Exercise 9.1: Drawing up a new compassionate formulation for your overeating*    214

Summary    218

**10   Motivating yourself to change**

The seven stages of change    219

Why think about the process of change?    222

Compassionate motivation    223

    *Exercise 10.1: What stage of change am I in and how can I move forward?*    225

    *Exercise 10.2: Recognizing the benefits and costs of overeating*    225

Improving your chances of success: planning for blocks
to change                                                               227

    *Exercise 10.3: Identifying practical problems*              228

    *Exercise 10.4: Overcoming practical problems*              228

Getting support to help you resolve overeating              230

    *Exercise 10.5: Identifying sources of help*              231

Compassionately managing setbacks                            232

Summary                                                                 233

**11   Working out what your body needs**

Looking after our physical needs                              235

What does your body need?                                      236

Moving towards balanced eating that meets your needs    240

Working out what you're eating now                          241

    *Exercise 11.1: Identifying difficulties in calorie estimating*   242

    *Exercise 11.2: My compassionate thoughts and actions for*   242
        *managing estimating my energy intake*

Working out your energy balance                              248

    *Exercise 11.3: Working out your own energy balance*   255

Summary                                                                 256

**12   Towards a new way of eating: the first steps**

The six-step programme: an outline                          257

    *Exercise 12.1: Planning to eat more regularly*          259

    *Exercise 12.2: Managing blocks to eating regularly*    264

Summary                                                                 273

**13   Towards a new way of eating: the final steps**

The benefits of meal planning                                274

Potential problems with meal planning                        275

*Exercise 13.1: Identifying potential problems with meal planning*  275

*Exercise 13.2: Learning to feel hunger and fullness*  288

*Exercise 13.3: Changing food associations*  291

*Exercise 13.4: Enjoying eating socially*  292

Putting it all together: caring for your body with compassion  293

Summary  297

**14  Compassionate letter writing**

Getting started  299

Setting the scene for compassionate letter writing  300

Steps to compassionate letter writing  301

*Exercise 14.1: Imagining offering compassion to yourself*  313

*Exercise 14.2: Finding your compassionate voice*  314

Making time to write your letter  315

Summary  317

**15  A compassionate focus on eating: final thoughts**

*Useful resources*  323

*References*  327

*Extra worksheets*  329

*Index*  364

# Introduction

We humans have always understood that compassion is very important for our well-being. Recent advances in scientific studies of compassion and kindness have greatly advanced our understanding of how compassionate qualities of the mind really do influence our brains, bodies and social relationships, as well as affecting our health and well-being. Yet despite this ancient wisdom and modern knowledge we live in an age that can make compassion for ourselves and others difficult. This is the world of the competitive edge, of achievement and desire, of comparison, dissatisfaction and criticism. Research has now revealed that such environments actually make us unhappier, and that mental ill-health is on the increase, especially in younger people. These issues are particularly pronounced in those of us who have difficulties with our eating habits and/or our weight. As Dr Goss helps us see, we are surrounded by a food industry that wants us to eat more and more, deliberately manipulating taste, texture and aesthetic appeal, and also by a culture that is highly critical of the overweight. Caught between the two, the more we criticize ourselves and feel down about our difficulties with eating, the more we eat. Learning compassion – particularly for ourselves – offers a path out of this cycle.

Another aspect of our society is a habit of attaching blame to people if they do not seem to come up to the mark or behave in prescribed ways. However, as Ken Goss makes clear, we can have significant difficulty with eating and weight through no fault of our own. We are a species on a long and continuing evolutionary journey. We didn't design our brains with their various capacities for emotions, like anxiety and anger, and their desires for sex or a lovely tasty meal – this is just how our brains are. Nor did we design our bodies to seek out foods high in fat, sugar and calorie content – that's just the way they've evolved. We developed few natural regulators in our minds to limit our intake of such foods because we didn't need them on the savannas of prehistoric Africa, where these foods are very scarce. Today, though, it is tricky when you can go into a supermarket and find highly manufactured foods that can light up our brains of 'wanting and appetites' like Christmas trees.

What are we to do, then? First, we can learn to pay attention to how our minds work and function, and become mindful and observant of the feelings that are associated with eating. Ken Goss shows in helpful detail how people have learned to pay attention to their feelings rather than simply reaching for the fridge.

If our relationship with ourselves is critical and harsh, then our inner worlds are not comfortable places to be in. Feeling ashamed, and being self-critical, self-condemning or even self-loathing can undermine our confidence, make us feel bad – and tempt us to eat more! In contrast, self-compassion is a way of being with ourselves in all our emotions, uncomfortable as they may be, without self-condemning and with support and encouragement. Research shows that the more compassionate we are towards ourselves, the happier we are, and the more resilient we are when faced with difficult events in our lives. In addition, we are better able to reach out to others for help, and more compassionate with other people too.

Compassion is sometimes viewed as being a bit soft or weak, letting your guard down and not trying hard enough. Quite the contrary. Compassion requires us to be open to and tolerate our painful feelings, to face up to our own difficulties and those of others. Compassion is not turning away from difficulty or discomfort, or trying to get rid of it. It is not a soft option. It requires courage, honesty and a commitment to do what we can to alleviate unhappiness and pain of all kinds. It teaches us to do things to and for ourselves that help us to flourish and take care of ourselves – not as a demand or requirement, but to enable us to live our lives more fully and contentedly.

In this book Ken Goss draws on his many years of experience heading the NHS eating disorders service in Coventry, UK. In particular he has developed compassion-focused therapy for people with eating disorders and disordered eating. Here he outlines a compassionate way of thinking about our evolved and complex relationships with food and provides a number of steps and exercises that enable you to develop a compassionate approach to those difficulties. You will learn about the nature of compassion and how to develop compassionate attention, compassionate thinking and compassionate behaviour. You will learn about the potential power of developing compassionate imagery and the compassionate sense of self, and how to use them when things get tough. Compassionate images can be either visual or aural (e.g. imagining a compassionate voice speaking to you when you need it), and can be especially useful in enabling us to get in touch with our internal compassionate feelings and desires.

The compassionate mind approach outlined here draws on many other well-developed approaches, including those of Eastern traditions such as Buddhism and Western therapeutic approaches such as the various cognitive behavioural therapies. Recognizing that one has a difficult, sometimes a love–hate relationship with food and eating, is a first step towards change; the next is to think about what would be helpful, followed by moving on with a programme of clear, practical steps towards change. This book provides such a programme. What a compassionate mind approach adds is that when you identify the steps, you begin to walk the path in a friendly, supportive, kind and encouraging way, recognizing that from time to time you will trip up, things will not go as you wish and you will have setbacks and relapses – but that every time kindness, compassion and support will help you through. You will learn to develop an inner voice that conveys a sense of understanding, encouragement and warmth for you. If, by the end of this book, you have learned only how to speak to yourself kindly, you will have gained a valuable skill.

Many people suffer silently and secretly with eating and weight – some ashamed of or angry with it, others sometimes fearful of it. Sadly, shame stops many of us from reaching out from help. But by opening your heart to compassion for your eating you can take the first steps towards dealing with it in a new way. Our compassionate wishes go with you on your journey.

Professor Paul Gilbert
August 2010

# Acknowledgements

My first thanks go to all those clients who have been willing to share their experience of overeating. Their insights have been invaluable, while their courage and commitment to learning ways to deal with their experiences and feelings have inspired my work for over twenty years.

This book would never have been written without the support and encouragement of Professor Paul Gilbert. I have had the privilege of working with Paul for almost my entire professional career. His influence has been profound in both my personal and my professional life. He has pioneered the development of compassion-focused therapy, and his commitment to developing, researching and promoting this new approach has moved compassion into the mainstream of scientific thinking and clinical practice. I will always remain grateful for his help and for encouraging me to take responsibility for bringing the developments I have made in working with people with eating disorders to a wider audience. Without his faith in my ability to complete this work, and his compassionate encouragement throughout the process of writing, I would never have finished.

I would like to thank my family, Gill, Adam and Tasha, for their patience and encouragement in completing this book. Books take time to grow, and this one has taken several years! It is my greatest hope that they will always experience compassion from others and from themselves.

Finally, I would like to thank you, the reader, for taking the time to consider a different way of dealing with food and eating. I hope it can help you to find new ways to care for yourself and manage the challenges of life.

# How to use this book

This book consists of two intertwined elements: an outline of the compassionate mind approach to human psychology, and specifically to our relationships with food, eating and our bodies; and a practical programme of staged tasks that will help you relate these ideas to your own life and your own habits, thoughts and feelings around food and eating.

Throughout the book from Chapter 5 onwards you will find exercises you can do and worksheets you can use to keep records. Try the exercises in your own time and at your own pace. Blank copies of the various worksheets are provided at the back of the book; you can photocopy as many of these as you need, and you may wish to adapt them to make them personal to you. You may also find it useful to have a notebook and pen with you as you work through the book so that you can make your own notes on things that you find particularly useful or challenging.

This book contains a lot of ideas, and on first reading it may seem to you that the prospect of change is too complex, difficult or overwhelming. The key is to go one step at a time: try things out for yourself, see what you can use, and if you only change one or two things, that's still helpful. Few of us follow manuals or recipes to the letter, if we're honest. But we also know that if we want to get fit, play the piano or learn a foreign language, the more we practise the better we'll get.

# 1 Understanding our relationship with food

Food can be a pleasure or a curse. Without it we die, and with too much we have a whole range of health problems. We eat for a host of reasons: because we're hungry, to be sociable, because we're miserable, or because we just like the taste and the pleasure of putting things in our mouth. We enjoy our food because of its tastes and textures. For most of us, chocolate cakes and ice creams are an awful lot more desirable than turnips and spinach. Unfortunately, the latter are much better for you. Although over half the world does not have enough to eat, many of us in the West have the opposite problem – managing the availability of relatively cheap and appetizing food. The abundance of easily accessible processed foods brings with it serious difficulties relating to how we manage our desire for food, and regulate our appetites and weight. In the modern Western world we are surrounded with enticements to buy and eat more. If we follow these cultural demands we are pretty likely to put on weight – but then we often become the target of moral and medical condemnation, feeling guilty or ashamed about our eating. Simply telling ourselves not to eat too much is not a great deal of help. Indeed, it tends to make things worse because we now feel depressed so we eat more to feel better. Sometimes it can feel as if you just can't win!

## What does a 'compassionate mind' approach mean?

Understanding this difficulty is actually the first step towards developing a compassionate approach to food and eating. When we look more closely at overeating we come to understand how complex it is, and to realize that it's not our fault that so many of us struggle to regulate our eating behaviour and weight. It turns out that our brains have evolved to be attracted to foods that are high in fat and sugar and our bodies have evolved to store excess energy (in the form of fat) for leaner times. Your brain is not really designed to regulate your eating, because for much of the time over which mammals have evolved it didn't need to: food was hard to find, so we had to make the most of it when it was available.

Once we give up blaming ourselves for the problems we have with our diets and our weight, we become less ashamed and more open to taking responsibility for finding ways to eat, and to exercise, that are appropriate and helpful for us. This is a hard task, and it's even more difficult to tackle it if we are swamped by self-critical feelings.

A compassionate mind approach, then, starts with understanding what we're up against. This means understanding how, and in what conditions, our brains evolved to give us certain desires and passions, and how modern environments can make life both easier for us in some ways and also very difficult in others.

## Understanding the problem: why we love to eat

Let's go back a million years or so and consider how our ancestors back then lived. They would have spent much of their time foraging for food, because it was usually in short supply and they were not as good at hunting as other meat-eating animals such as lions, wolves and hyenas. Foraging animals eat as often as they can, because food is often hard to find. Seeking it out requires a lot of time and energy, and foragers are constantly on the move. Most accounts of *our* ancestors suggest that this was the way they lived for many thousands of years.

In this environment, our brains did not evolve mechanisms for self-restraint because they did not need them: our eating was constrained by the relative shortage of food and our foraging habits. We evolved for the *'see-food' diet*: 'see food and eat it'! Actually, many mammals are like this – you may recognize the tendency in your family dog. It's not our fault that our brains and bodies did not evolve with effective mechanisms for self-restraint in eating; but the fact that they didn't can make life very difficult for us in the modern world, where many of us have easy access to cheap, nutritious food and tend to be far less active than in former times.

What about the food itself? Well, most of the food our ancestors would have foraged for would have been pretty low in calories, and so they needed to eat a lot of it. It is true that we also became hunters of meat and could bring down large game, particularly when we operated in (mostly male) teams. However, hunting tends to be a pretty hit-and-miss affair: even the most successful carnivores actually make a meal out of only about one in ten of their intended prey. So although meat was an important part of our ancestors' diet, for the most part they would have relied on nuts, berries, root vegetables and other plants: meat and fish would have been a bonus!

Looking at groups around the world who have a more basic way of life than us in the developed West, we find that they tend not to be big meat-eaters. Their diet consists mainly of foods that can be gathered – often by women – roots, nuts and vegetables. Also, many plants evolved fruits and seeds that were palatable to herbivores, so that they would eat them and spread the seeds; thus when ripe they were sweet-tasting, as a result of a high sugar content that made them both appetizing and naturally high in calorie (energy) content. In fact, the sugary taste is how we know they are ripe: plants that are poisonous or not ripe tend to have a sour taste. Therefore, we evolved with a sweet tooth!

Other energy-dense foods (like fish or meat) tend to have higher fat and protein contents. They were harder to obtain but keep us fuller for longer compared to roots, vegetables and berries. A diet rich in meat and fish thus gave hunters an evolutionary advantage in times of famine. In more bountiful times it also meant that, rather than having to constantly forage, humans had time between hunting expeditions for thinking and making things. This led to an explosion in human development, as we became toolmakers and planners.

So our desire for high-fat and high-sugar foods, together with an increasingly intelligent brain with which to find them, and interest in sharing them with other group members, gave us a huge evolutionary advantage. However, as these foods were in short supply, we never had to develop the means to restrain our appetites or our weight – we simply didn't need the brain that would do this! We needed the *see-food-and-eat-it* (particularly sweet or fatty food) brain. The trouble is that now, for a relatively small proportion of the human population – those who live in rich industrialized societies, where sweet and fatty foods are plentiful and cheap – the see-food-and-eat-it brain is no longer helpful. Indeed, it is becoming a major problem for many of us, who are eating much more than our ancestors and taking much less exercise, and developing unhealthy eating habits and becoming overweight as a result.

To make matters worse, we – like most animals – also evolved to be an energy-conserving species. This means that when we have eaten enough to meet our energy needs we will tend to become less active. We only get more active when we need to go and find more food because we are hungry. So we have an inherent tendency to become couch potatoes!

There is another interesting aspect to our story. We don't know exactly when humans evolved, but the process began around two million years ago. What we do know is that along the way humans became a strongly cooperative species, wanting to share a whole range of resources and information with one another. Indeed, language would not have evolved had we not taken an interest in communicating with each other. Hunting relied on social cooperation and the subsequent sharing of the meal. The most successful hunters (those lions, wolves and hyenas) are very sociable within their own groups; they follow very specific rules about eating after a kill to ensure that those who are most valuable to the group all receive a share. We think that these habits also developed among our human ancestors, and so getting food and sharing it became strongly linked to our social lives. Even today, one of the most important ways we entertain each other is to cook for each other, and we love going out for meals together. In many non-Western societies we see the same basic preference for eating together and sharing food. For the most part eating is a highly social event, associated with pleasurable feelings of togetherness and security.

Being fed has always been a comforting experience for humans. Breast feeding has calmed and soothed babies and young children the world over for millennia. Feeding can be soothing – understandably, as it signals the physical closeness of a care-giver and the safeness that this offers. Eating in social groups has also been with us for thousands of years; and still eating together and sharing our food solidifies our relationships with others. Where resources are scarce, it helps us manage their use effectively. When they are more plentiful, we want to share high-quality food, to be seen as generous and as good cooks. Thus eating together can be a source of both pleasure and social comfort. So there is nothing wrong with deriving comfort from food; indeed, it is a very natural way of being soothed by others. However, at most times in human history the comfort derived from food was self-limiting: mothers can only produce so much milk, and social groups often struggled to find enough to eat.

Our natural preference for sweet foods can easily be used to train us to behave in certain ways, and such foods may actually soothe us (as we will explore in Chapter 3). The link between sweet foods and rewards, or even approval – 'being a good boy or girl' – is made early if sweets are given as a reward for behaving in a particular way. For example, imagine you are in a crowded supermarket, your child is crying and you know you will be stuck in the queue for a least another twenty minutes . . . It is easy to see how we could end up giving them a sweet, both to take their mind off their distress and to comfort them, and of course parents learn that it can work! So they do it again and again. So what do we do when we are upset as adults? We do what we have learned to do, of course – where's that chocolate? What do we do when we feel we want a reward or want to celebrate? Yep – go for the food and drink, the good night out or a raid on the fridge. We sometimes find that people with eating problems as adults were often soothed with food as children, rather than with hugs or by talking things through and learning how to manage emotions. Indeed, some people are not aware of the link between their emotions and eating.

Of course, until recently in most parts of the world, cakes, chocolate bars, chips and crisps weren't available to be used by parents as treats and pacifiers. But today, from the day we are born to the day we die, food is linked in our minds to enjoyment, treats, celebrating, socializing, having friends, caring, calming difficult emotions and a sense of deserving – and much more. It is unlikely that there has been any time in our history where food has had such complex and multiple associations and meanings.

In a world in which we all have less and less time to care for ourselves and others, where many of us are working in two or more jobs just to keep up, food (and of course drink) has become one way in which we have learned to reward ourselves, manage our feelings or comfort those around us. It's not surprising, then, that those of us who have grown up in the past century have increasingly associated food with comfort and soothing of distress on the one hand, and also with rewards and having a good time on the other.

We have to be honest, too, in acknowledging that sometimes our problems with food relate to quite complicated emotional difficulties. We know that some children are relatively neglected or come from difficult and abusive families. Having never really felt loved or connected or worthy, they can spend a lot of time as adults trying to cope with difficult emotions with roots in their childhoods. Food can get caught up in all that. Someone who tended to binge-eat once told me that it was like a rebellion: she could do it, and no one could stop her. It was also a way of keeping down painful feelings of loneliness and anger which at times came close to overwhelming to her. 'Food,' she said, 'thinking about it, imagining it, planning to eat and enjoying it – is a way of distracting myself from the pain in my life. Problem is, after I finish bingeing I feel disgusted with myself and so the whole cycle starts up again, fuelled by anger that I can't do anything about.'

Some people struggling to cope with emotional difficulties in this way develop serious eating disorders such as bulimia or anorexia. These are usually best tackled with professional support, though self-help certainly can have a part to play. However, many people who do not develop these grave illnesses still struggle with their eating habits, and often feel angry, ashamed and anxious as a result. If you're one of them, this book is for you and all those like you – from those who just overdo it at Christmas to habitual binge-eaters, from those who raid the fridge when they're upset to those who find it hard to stop eating once they've started. If any of these descriptions ring a bell, and if you want to develop a healthy relationship with food and to do so in a way that will care for your real needs, both physical and emotional, then this book is for you.

It is important to recognize and have compassion for the complexity of our relationship with food, eating and weight. Sometimes we lose control of our eating because we're going through a very unhappy time in our life, and our relationship with food is caught up in all that. If we are gentle with ourselves and kind to ourselves, if we recognize and accept this complexity and the pain that can be hidden behind the 'food problem', we have a better chance of working with these issues. All the time keep in mind that if you're struggling with food there are reasons for it that are to do with how *all* humans have evolved, which is hardly something you can blame yourself for! Once you come to understand this, and then free yourself from the shame and the blame that so often go with overeating, you can then move on to think about what's really going to help you; what's really in your best interests and how you can look after yourself and urge yourself on to be your very best – and yes, you do deserve that, even if a little voice in your head says, 'Oh no you don't.'

## The perils of modern societies and supermarkets

As the human brain evolved, so did its intelligence, and it wasn't far along the road of human evolution that we worked out that you don't need to look for food – you can make food come to you. Humans became farmers, planting our crops rather than going out to gather them, and herding and breeding livestock rather than roaming the plains looking for animals to kill. No longer did we have to spend our time firing arrows that missed the buffalo by a mile and getting back to the camp exhausted; we simply went to the pen and knocked one on the head. It's not quite Tesco's or Wal-Mart down the road yet, but we were on our way. Over time, of course, barter and then money came into the equation and food became a commodity to be traded like many others – and so, over the past few thousand years, we have trudged down the trail towards modern capitalist societies where we get our food in a totally different way from how we evolved to find and eat it. It's all much easier, of course; but it's created new problems.

Modern Western societies have allowed industries to exploit that old evolutionary 'see-food-and-eat-it' drive in our brains, and those deep and powerful associations between food, pleasure and security. The food industry spends billions of pounds artificially enhancing the taste, texture and look of foods to tempt us to buy them *and* to associate them in our minds with having a good time, surrounded by happy people such as family and friends. Sometimes foods are advertised as 'secret pleasures', but usually the subliminal message is that eating high-fat and high-sugar foods goes with social pleasures such as enjoying family outings or parties.

Not only are the foods themselves tempting to our see-food-and-eat-it brain, the ways they are packaged and displayed in supermarkets are designed to tempt you even more. Supermarkets employ psychologists to help them find the most effective ways to do this. For example, that smell of freshly baked bread stimulates your appetite, and the sight of the cream cakes and two-for-one offers encourages you to buy more than you might have planned. Sweets are placed near check-out tills where stressed shoppers, accompanied by bored children, can easily reach them.

Another worrying development is the increasingly widespread use in farming and food processing of a wide range of fertilizers, chemicals and preservatives. We're not entirely sure what many of these substances do. There is increasing evidence that some preservatives can have significant effects, for example on children's moods. We simply don't know the effects on people who overeat, especially if they eat a lot of processed foods, and are taking in lots of these chemicals. Is it affecting their moods?

Of course, this isn't to cast supermarkets as out-and-out villains: they're not deliberately trying to cause problems, and they also provide us with good-quality fresh food, including a wide range of fruit and vegetables that even a few years ago were not readily available to most people. However, while they're not deliberately trying to cause problems, they're not in business to help us manage our eating either. They are in business to provide what we are prepared to buy, and to entice us to buy and consume as much of it as they can. It is only sensible to recognize that the food industry is not set up to provide us with the healthiest foods, or to help us limit our diets sensibly: it is set up to provide us with as much as we will buy of the foods we will pay for, and we evolved to have a preference for sweet and fatty foods.

Modern Western societies have a rather damaging tendency to blame the individual for problems that are in fact side-effects of our new ways of living, and to see them as our individual, rather than collective, responsibility to sort out. But it's really difficult for most of us to understand how our brains and bodies, which evolved in a very different environment over many thousands of years, are responding to the demands and enticements of a modern world that has come into being over mere decades – or at the most a couple of centuries. So, rather than seeing the problem clearly, we as individuals get squeezed in the middle between the pressures to overeat and the warnings that we shouldn't – and it is all too easy for us to end up taking the blame for problems we didn't cause. As a result we end up feeling inadequate, ashamed, helpless and hopeless in managing our eating and weight. These feelings in turn completely undermine our ability to cope with our difficulties. So it is not surprising that we turn to the diet industry for ready-made answers and hope, and then blame ourselves yet again when these solutions do not work.

## Our need for compassion

It doesn't take long, really, does it, to begin to understand the problems we face and to see that in trying to deal with our eating habits we are actually dealing with complex relationships between our current diets, our weight and our feelings about ourselves? It is all a bit tricky. We may eat because we are happy, because we're just enjoying eating and/or because we're celebrating (speaking personally, feel-good times are actually my danger times); we may eat because everybody else is eating and we just go along with that; we may eat because we feel unhappy, miserable and alone; and we may eat to distract us from the unhappiness and difficulties in our lives.

As I've already said, our compassionate journey towards a healthy relationship with food must begin with a clear understanding that this relationship is a complex one. The way our brains have evolved has set us up to have problems that our modern society has simply added to – and we're not responsible for either ancient evolution or modern society! The moment you begin to move away from self-blaming and self-criticism, to take shame out of the complicated web of feelings associated with eating, you will be free to think about how to help yourself in a more compassionate and responsible way. Rather than fighting against temptations, you can learn to work with them.

The key message of this book, then, is this: your overeating is not your fault, but you *can* take responsibility for it – and gain control over it, too, *if* you are supportive and kind to yourself along the way. As the book progresses – and particularly in Chapter 4 – we will investigate more thoroughly what being 'kind' to yourself means. An advert on television may tell you that being nice to yourself is treating yourself to cream cakes and boxes of chocolates – but if you eat too many of them, you may be giving yourself health problems. It's much kinder, actually – much more compassionate – to learn how to acknowledge and respond to your real needs, rather than being easy prey to tempters who really just want you to spend money on their products!

Physical and psychological health professionals, too, need to understand this message very clearly. I see many clients who tell me that their conversations with professionals have left them feeling rather ashamed and criticized. There has been an undertone that overweight is simply about greed or laziness, about lack of willpower, lack of control, lack of effort – well, lack of everything, really. Having been shamed, blamed and stigmatized, of course people then simply turn off, tune out, get depressed, withdraw and take solace in the only thing that can be guaranteed to give them a little pleasure – food! They may also feel a certain amount of anger and rebelliousness – one person who had been told off by a professional went back home and thought, 'How rude you are – how unkind – and how much you don't understand me – well, to hell with you, then,' and raided the fridge.

## Moving away from moral judgements about eating

Most of us who overeat will diet at some point as a way to manage our weight and/or our appetite for certain foods. All weight-loss diets aim to restrict our eating below the level of energy that our body needs, but we may also try to limit the types of food we eat because they are seen as in some way unhealthy for us. For example, until relatively recently diabetics were required to cut out all sugary foods to manage their condition (although more recently these very strict eating rules have been relaxed as the medical profession has recognized that such a restrictive diet is not usually necessary and that clients find it very difficult to maintain anyway).

Anyone who has tried to diet will be only too well aware that television programmes, magazines and diet books are full of conflicting advice and pseudoscience. The diet industry is worth billions of pounds worldwide, and hardly a week goes by without some new fad or diet being launched, or some celebrity telling us how they lost 10 pounds in a week! And yet, despite all this advice, the Western world is plagued by obesity and obesity-related diseases, by eating disorders and eating problems – some of which can have profound psychological and physical consequences. With so many conflicting messages, we can feel damned if we do diet and damned if we don't.

Many of these diets and diet programmes also contain hidden messages – for example, that if you have a weight problem then it's because there is something wrong *with you*. How many actually tell you that you have been surrounded by foods that are deliberately made difficult to resist by the food industry? They imply that if you are a reasonable person you will *want* to lose weight by controlling your eating; so if you don't control your eating, or you struggle to lose weight, then somehow you must be an unreasonable or weak-willed person! A lot of diets also imply that with a little willpower – and, of course, *their* diet – actually controlling your eating and losing weight is really not so difficult. Therefore, if you're finding it difficult and tough going, if you have a few successes but then put the weight back on again, that is again because there's a problem with *you*. No wonder many people who are overweight or struggling with their eating feel ashamed!

There are even competitive reality TV programmes that follow members of the public and celebrities as they struggle to manage their weight. These entice us to pass judgement on those who are succeeding or failing in their battle with food and the scales. People are asked to leave – are *rejected* – if they don't lose as much as others, or seem to be not putting enough effort in. We don't yet know for sure what the effects of this are on participants' self-esteem or confidence, but it seems highly likely they aren't positive ones. These rather cruel programmes feed – and feed on – our fascination with people's struggles, but also invite us to treat those 'contestants' who don't make it at best dismissively and at worst with contempt and ridicule. We are not encouraged to feel sympathy for them, to understand the complex reasons for their relationship with food and their bodies, to hear of (maybe) the stories of early emotional neglect or the sadness and loneliness of a bullied childhood. Nor are we invited to follow the longer-term journey that these people take – including those who 'win' but regain weight at a later date.

Current evidence suggests that only one dieter in twenty who loses a significant amount of weight will maintain this loss in the long term. Even people taking part in research trials, with a high degree of professional support, are unlikely to lose more than 4–10 kilograms and maintain this for at least a year. If we are overweight, only a moderate amount of weight loss (approximately 5–10 per cent) is necessary to provide some improvement in health, and anything more than this tends to be impossible to maintain in the long run. Yet most diet programmes promote a far higher level of weight loss that this and suggest that the results can be maintained for ever if only we follow their advice.

Television is entertainment, and these programmes need winners and losers, heroes and villains, to maintain the drama of the story. Like the old Roman gladiatorial games, they manipulate our feelings, discouraging us from sympathizing with the losers – after all, the very format is not designed for us to have compassion for *everybody* in the programme: if we did, there would simply be no drama. However, this way of viewing the world also fits in with, and reinforces, our cultural perceptions of those who struggle with eating, and often even our own feelings about our relationship with food and our bodies. Winner or loser; hero or villain; triumphant achiever or abject failure; compassion and sympathy or contempt and ridicule: these are just some of the complex oppositions that those who have dieted may recognize in the relationship they have with their eating and their bodies. No wonder such programmes make compulsive viewing for so many people.

Of course, anyone who has ever been on a diet (and this includes me) will know that losing weight, and keeping it off, is actually pretty tricky.

However, when we run into obstacles in our quest to control our eating and weight it is common for us to blame ourselves, and this tendency is supported by many diet regimes. For example, negative attitudes and moral judgements about food and eating are often reflected in the language used: in some diets, certain foods are seen as a 'sin' or a 'treat'; in others, certain foods are given 'points', values that are to be earned. Being weighed in front of others at a slimming club can be seen as a supportive gesture, but also as a way of putting pressure on participants through the potential for ritual humiliation in front of the group. Many of these diets and clubs focus on successes with weight loss, holding them up as positive motivation – but what about those who feel too ashamed to reach out for help, or who wander off because they feel they are failing?

I work with many people who have come to see eating as bad, or a sin, or something they have to earn, rather than something their body needs to do in order to function; people who report binge-eating after being weighed publicly, either as a treat for their success in losing weight or as a punishment for not losing anything, or not losing enough. A compassionate mind approach to managing our weight needs to move away from these moral judgements and their inherent criticism of our need and desire to eat. It requires us to support the changes in eating behaviour we wish to make without attacking and criticizing ourselves when we struggle, as we inevitably will when finding ways to manage our see-food-and-eat-it brain and complex emotional system. We also need to learn to focus more on our health and well-being and less on the feelings of success or competition that can be associated with seeing the numbers on the scales go down, and to learn other ways to feel a sense of success and to be comforted when we are distressed. This means putting food back in its place, as an important and enjoyable part of our lives, something that can be shared with others, and not a threat to our health or sense of personal well-being.

## How this books works

In this book we will explore some of the contradictions involved in trying to change our weight, and some of the obstacles we meet. This will include looking at how our bodies have evolved to eat and drink and to regulate our appetite. We will also look at how our body manages our attempts to eat too much or too little food. We will see how, if we attempt to alter our body's natural mechanisms for managing our shape and weight, this can have a significant effect on our ability to let our body maintain its weight. We will explore how to find out what our personal healthy weight is – and this doesn't mean an 'ideal weight' according to weight charts and diet books (whose prescriptions, by the way, change quite dramatically over the years), but a weight that is ideal for us to function healthily.

Sadly, many of us never really discover what our naturally healthy weight is. There are a number of reasons for this, including the recent availability of calorie-rich foods, our generally more sedentary lifestyle, changes in the way we eat (including eating 'on the go' rather than savouring and enjoying mealtimes) and an increasing link between eating, or not eating, and regulating our emotional life.

I hope that as you read through this book you will find ways to get back in touch with your body. You will learn to respond to the need for food and drink and to manage some of the complex challenges that our new ways of producing and consuming food pose to letting our body reach its naturally healthy weight. As you discover more about the complex links between food and our emotional life, and find ways to disentangle the two, you can let your body do what it is designed to do (keeping healthy) and find other ways to manage your thoughts and feelings instead of using food to do this.

Self-criticism is incredibly common in people who diet. This is often one of the most important factors in lowering our mood and isolating ourselves from others. Moreover, constantly criticizing ourselves when our diets don't work, or when we break the rules we set ourselves around what we should eat, when we should eat, how we should eat and why we should eat, is almost bound to lead to failure in our attempts to manage our eating. The new understandings and skills you will learn in this book will help you develop a new relationship with food and eating, free you from unhelpful self-criticism, and increase your chance of letting your body find a weight that is healthy and sustainable for you. You might like just now to think about whether you tend to criticize yourself a lot, particularly around issues of size, shape, weight and eating. If you do, then this book is probably going to be useful to you.

The key to the approach set out in this book is learning compassion towards ourselves and others. As I've said already, compassion begins with understanding, and the early chapters of this book aim to help you come to a better understanding of how our brains and bodies work. This is not another diet book, although it will help you find ways to manage your food intake and energy output that are more in tune with your body's needs. Instead, it offers you a different approach to learning to live in a complex body, in a world it was not evolved to live in, with a mind that also hasn't really evolved to deal with all these problems in the first place! It could help you find new ways to deal with the very complex challenges we all face as human beings, particularly in a rich country where food is plentiful. These challenges include:

- to learn to regulate our eating in a way that is best for both our physical health and psychological well-being;

- to be able to accept and live comfortably with the notion that there are normal variations in human size, shape, and weight, and that the shape we might wish to be might not be the size or shape we are biologically designed to be;

- to be able to accept and value human beings, including ourselves, regardless of their, and our, weight and shape;

- to be able to manage our feelings without using food as our main or only way of coping with distress.

Many chapters contain exercises to help you explore these issues and make sense of your own relationship with food and eating. You may well come to think, as I have, that our bodies are pretty tricky things and that managing them can be hard work; but I hope you will also come to believe, as I have, that it is possible to do so – without constantly criticizing ourselves or feeling under pressure, and without 'going on a diet'. We will explore a different approach to eating that involves learning to respond to our body's needs. This is more likely to lead to long-term weight change and stability than following any of the myriads of dietary fads, which although initially appealing usually end up in failure.

In Chapter 2, we will explore 'set-point theory': the idea that your body evolved to keep you at a healthy weight (your 'set point') if you feed it enough energy on a regular basis. We will also explore the various ways in which you can affect your body's set point, including eating too much or too little, your eating pattern, other substances you take into your body, and of course your emotional life.

In Chapter 3 we will explore the complex relationship between eating and feeling – how eating relates to our thoughts, emotions and relationships. We will also explore the impact that dieting, or denying ourselves foods, can have on our feelings, and how in turn this can lead us to feeling self-critical and ashamed.

In Chapter 4 we will explore the meaning of compassion in relation to our overall emotional and mental makeup, and in relation to our attitudes to food. We will explore some of the mindsets that lead us to overeat, and consider how a more compassionate mindset can help us manage our relationship with food and eating, and our emotional life, in a more effective way.

Chapter 5 introduces the first exercises, as we begin work on developing our 'compassionate mind', particularly through the use of compassionate imagery. Many people who overeat find this difficult, but, as we will see, through gentle practice and persistence we can train our minds to work in this different way.

We expand on these skills in Chapter 6, concentrating on developing the skills of self-compassion. These include new ways of activating the 'sooth-ing system' that we all have in our brains to help manage your feelings without needing food. We will also explore ways to manage when your feelings become overwhelming, and the benefits of learning to tolerate these feelings so that you can come to understand them without resorting immediately to eating more than you need. Finally, we will explore new ways of thinking and acting from a self-compassionate perspective that can help you move away from the mindsets and patterns of behaviour that so often lead to overeating.

In the later chapters of this book, we will work on understanding how your overeating has developed and what keeps it going now. Chapter 7 outlines the compassionate mind approach to understanding the influences on your overeating, including the key threats it may have helped you to deal with, and how the unintended consequences of overeating may have made you likely to carry on overeating. Chapter 8 provides you with some skills for exploring your overeating in the here and now – in particular, using diaries to help you become more mindful of what, why and how you eat, as well as of the things that help you to avoid overeating. Chapter 9 brings all this information together to help you develop your own personal 'formulation' of how overeating works for you, so that you can use it as a basis for helping resolve overeating for good.

The next few chapters are all about changing the way you relate to food and your feelings. We begin Chapter 10 by looking at the process that we all go through, in one way or another, when making changes in our lives, and how this is likely to affect the changes you will make in tackling overeating. It also provides exercises to help you explore, maintain and increase your motivation, and to help you manage setbacks with compassion.

In Chapter 11 we explore how to work out what your body needs in terms of energy and nutrition, so that you can use this as a basis for changing your eating. In Chapter 12 we outline the steps to a healthy relationship with food and eating based on and maintained with compassion, starting with eating more regularly and managing foods that can trigger overeating. In Chapter 13 we build upon this foundation to help you plan to meet your nutritional needs, as you learn to recognize and respond to feeling hungry and full, to care for your body – and, finally, actually to enjoy eating!

Chapter 14 brings together all the new understanding and skills you have learned in developing self-compassion and working on overeating using an exercise called 'compassionate letter writing'. Chapter 15 sets out a brief summary of the key points of this approach. At the end of the book is a section of 'Useful resources' that may be valuable as you work through this book and in the future.

I have used examples of a number of clients in the book. You will meet Jane, David, Alison and Kerry as we go along. These are fictitious characters, but their histories and the problems they face are typical of many people I have worked with. None of them is based on any particular person, but have been developed to help you explore particular mindsets that can drive overeating.

This book is designed for the majority of us who overeat, and many people will be able to work through it happily and productively on their own. You may, however, find that you want some more support to help you tackle overeating. I have written the book with this in mind, so that you can use it on your own, with the help of a friend or in collaboration with a professional therapist. Also, if you are pregnant or have a serious physical illness it would be a good idea to consult a physician or dietitian as well as reading the book, as the broad guidelines about your energy needs may not be specific enough for your particular circumstances.

If your overeating is accompanied by feeling very depressed, if you deliberately vomit or use laxatives to help you manage your feelings about eating or your size and shape, or if you hurt yourself in other ways, you may need to seek professional help rather than use this book on its own. It is also important to note that if you are significantly underweight (if your body mass index (BMI) is under 18 – see page 29 for how to work this out), then you should seek medical support, either through your GP or from a professionally trained therapist. You can use some of the websites in the 'Useful resources' section to help you find advice.

As you work through this book, you will discover various examples of the complex relationship that we can have with food. We will explore how a compassionate mind approach can help you to understand your relationship with food, to move towards a non-dieting life, and gradually to accept yourself for who you are, including your size and shape. Moreover, it will help you move towards a place in the world where you can find fulfilment and happiness, and to cope with life's inevitable ups and downs without the highs and lows depending mainly on your relationship with food and your body.

# 2 Making sense of overeating, part 1: how our bodies work

## When survival skills backfire

As we saw in Chapter 1, our 'see-food-and-eat-it' brain gave us a massive evolutionary advantage in times of unpredictability, shortage or famine. So we have a body that is very good at storing energy (as fat, muscle and glycogen) and able to survive for weeks at a time with a poor food supply – though some people's bodies do this more easily than others. Indeed, our body can even boost its immune system during periods of famine by absorbing essential minerals from our bones. Our body helps us survive until food becomes available by slowing down our reproductive system and the rate at which we burn energy. It even gives us a natural high to help us manage the distress caused by being hungry: this gives us an extra burst of energy and stops us sleeping until we find the next available food source. People who diet can become somewhat addicted to this 'high'.

These remarkable survival skills first became potentially problematic when we moved from nomadic hunter-gatherer groups into agricultural economies. It then became a little easier to obtain a more regular supply of protein (from the meat of domestic animals or products from them such as milk, eggs or cheese). All the same, even in these early economies food supplies could still be unreliable as they depended to a large extent on nature, and so our evolved body still provided us with an evolutionary advantage.

The problems that we face now with eating habits and obesity only really emerged as we became more efficient at producing reliable and sustainable supplies of energy-dense and good-tasting food. As this happened, over the past 200 years, we have moved away from the diet we evolved to eat (primarily fruit and vegetables, with a small amount of protein from fish and meat) to one of highly processed protein and carbohydrate with only a relatively small proportion of fruit and vegetables; and at the same time we have significantly reduced the energy we use in day-to-day life.

As we saw in Chapter 1, we also evolved with a sweet tooth and a strong disgust response to food that might be contaminated or poisonous. Experiments with rats and humans clearly show that when good-tasting foods are available we tend to prefer them over foods that are bland – and we tend to eat more of them than we actually need. One of the consequences of eating sweet or sugary food is that it forces our body to increase production of a hormone called insulin, which is designed to 'sweep up' excess glucose in the blood. Once the extra insulin has gone to work, the level of sugar in the blood – known as our 'blood sugar level' – drops, and our body interprets this as us being hungry. The longer this cycle goes on for, the more likely we are to want to eat more food than we need, and the more likely it is that this will be stored as fat. It may take several more thousands of years for our bodies to evolve further to make it easier for us to regulate our eating. In the meantime we need to learn to manage our body and brain. This chapter and the next one are designed to provide you with the information you need to begin to do this, and in particular to help you manage the complex relationship between your emotions, body shape, weight and eating.

## Body issues

Although we all share an evolutionary history it is pretty obvious that we are not all the same. There are lots of ways in which we differ – for example, in height, hair colour, sporting talent and intellectual abilities. It is important to recognize that our bodies are not all the same when it comes to eating and weight gain, either. There are several important differences that we need to take into account when we consider these issues.

The ease with which we put on weight is linked to basic physiology. For example, there are cells in your body called 'brown fat cells', which regulate how much fat you lay down. Some ethnic groups tend to put on weight faster than others because their bodies are better adapted to survive in environments where food is scarce. We all know people who seem to be able to eat loads but do not put on weight. Some of these will have a faster metabolic rate, so they tend to burn the food they consume more quickly than others; some are more active – even when resting, they fidget more! –

which both increases their metabolic rate and means they are using up more energy than people who are less active.

How easily we are satisfied by food also seems to vary between individuals. Some people, even when they are physically full, don't seem to experience the feeling of fullness. Many of us still feel able to put in a little bit more, having just an extra biscuit or bit of cheese. But for some people it's more serious: they are constantly hungry. The scientific reasons for this are still being investigated and there remains much to learn about hunger, appetite and craving regulation.

As we've already seen, regulating our eating isn't just a matter of will-power, as many diet gurus try to tell us: but yes, there are some people who seem to find it easier to control their desires than others. Why this should be so is also still a matter of scientific debate. We do know, however, that there are many things that can undermine willpower – for example, a lack of opportunities to learn to cope with our feelings, or unhelpful rules about how and what we are 'allowed' to eat. So although there are probably biological reasons why some people find it easier than others to keep control of their eating, psychological studies also suggest that we can learn to develop willpower by creating helpful conditions for our efforts.

It's important to note, then, that the differences between us in terms of appetite and weight gain, our ability to recognize when we're full and even our willpower are in large part biologically determined, and so out of our hands. We may be able to learn to manage them differently, but we are not responsible for how and why they occurred in the first place.

Different cultures find different body shapes and sizes attractive. There are cultures where women seek to put on weight because plumpness signals possession of resources and status. Sumo wrestlers try desperately to put on weight because this is culturally attractive and gives them advantage in the wrestling ring. There is nothing intrinsically attractive or unattractive in being large. However, in most Western cultures slimness is now the culturally desired shape for women, and a flat stomach and well-defined muscles are the desired shape for men.

Researchers have wondered why so much emphasis is placed upon on slimness in our society. There are potentially many reasons. One is that slimness and a high hip-to-waist ratio has come to indicate youth and health. There has certainly been an extensive change in preferred body shapes in the past fifty years. For example, the most widely admired film stars of the 1950s were women such as Jayne Mansfield and Marilyn Monroe, with notably curvaceous bodies (a low hip-to-waist ratio). These are very different figures from those of more recent pinup models such as Twiggy or Kate Moss. These almost prepubescent images highlight the competition to present oneself not only as thin but also as young – and indeed, considerable fortunes are spent on trying to make our bodies appear young. Interestingly, however, most men actually prefer larger women, and some researchers think this drive for thinness is more to do with women competing among themselves than with competition to please or attract men. There is an old saying that 'the men watch the women: the women watch each other'.

This competing to show ourselves to be slim *and* young-looking has arisen largely within capitalist societies in the past fifty years. It's difficult to find any other culture or time in history when this was so. Why should it have happened here and now? There is no doubt that it has been driven partly by clever advertising to operate on people's anxieties about social accept-ance. We live in a society that has become highly focused on how people look – which includes facial appearance, body size and clothes. So, again, a drive for a slim and young-looking body shape is partly linked to social and cultural definitions of what is attractive – and these in turn both feed off and are fed by consumer industries whose business is selling things.

Although the diet and fashion industries are very largely aimed at women, men have not escaped this cultural onslaught on body size and shape. Again, if you look at stars of the 1950s, very few have a Brad Pitt physique. Many of Mr Pitt's contemporaries, however, do – and many more men today would like to. (I had to give up on that idea ages ago!)

Men and women alike, if we cannot meet these goals we often feel inferior and ashamed, and fearful of being rejected; so we push ourselves to change our eating habits and our bodies to get closer to what we *think* is the 'ideal'.

And when – as is so often the case – we can't reach our unrealistic goals, we can also become very self-critical.

## Health issues

More pressure to eat less and weigh less has come from an entirely different source. Medical science has recently shown that there is a link between weight and health. People with a body mass index above a certain level are more likely to suffer from significant difficulties with blood pressure, vulnerability to diabetes, pressure on joints and so forth. Indeed, some of the health problems associated with being excessively overweight can be tragic. On the face of it, it's hard to argue with the message that we should avoid being overweight if it's doing us physical harm. But part of the problem with this message is that it comes with an associated idea that healthy is *morally* good and unhealthy is *morally* bad. So, if we are putting on weight because we can't control our eating or are eating an unhealthy diet, then there is something bad about *us*. This rather accusatory approach is reflected in the number of television programmes about losing weight where overweight people are targeted. In some cases, too, there are class undertones, with barely disguised suggestions that working-class people have poor diets because they are somehow lazy or can't be bothered to eat 'properly'. Again, all too often concerns about the consequences of being overweight, whether based on medical or commercial motives, have come to be increasingly associated with shame and problems of self-control.

Increasingly, a healthy lifestyle is seen as a matter of choice and failure to adopt one as shameful and weak. Smokers and drinkers who put themselves at risk are often the targets of shaming attacks by others, including the government and health professionals. Indeed, some in the medical profession have even debated whether treatment should be withheld from such individuals because resources are scarce and, they argue, should not be 'squandered' on people who don't 'look after themselves'. People with weight problems can similarly run into difficulties if their doctors feel that they are not making enough effort to control their weight. Many of my clients have stories to tell about health professionals who have not been very sympathetic to their struggle. And yet there is plenty of evidence that it is really difficult to lose weight and keep it off in the long term, and that one doesn't need to lose very much weight to become healthy – even if one still doesn't conform to social ideals.

It is hard not to feel as if you are caught between two worlds – one that tells you cream cakes are 'naughty but nice' and hires popular football stars to advertise crisps, and one populated by people in white coats who imply there is something morally suspect about you if you can't control your weight. No wonder so many people struggle with eating and weight, and criticize themselves when they cannot exert perfect control over their appetite or desire for food!

It's also important to keep in mind that most of us in the modern Western world rarely use our bodies for the things they evolved to do, namely the various kinds of physical activity that filled up the vast majority of most people's lives from hunter-gatherer times to the middle ages. Over the past 200 years our working life has become more sedentary, and manual work has become the exception rather than the norm. We are far more likely to travel by car or public transport than by foot or bicycle as our homes are further from our jobs; and the fear of harm has meant that our children are less likely to walk to school, play outside, or even take part in some sports at school or in clubs, while curriculum pressures have all too often resulted in less and less time being given to formal and informal physical activity in the school week. There is now a real concern about the lack of physical activity that we and our children take, but it's only recently that our governments have woken up to the problem and tried to introduce schemes to encourage us to be more active.

But again, even if we want to be physically active, it can be difficult to fit exercise around our working and family lives. Cultural changes and constraints are no more our fault than our biological makeup is; and yet they do pose significant problems in how we manage our bodies.

I'm not suggesting for a moment that we should ignore these health issues or brush them under the carpet. Indeed, focusing on what helps you flourish is central to compassion focused therapy. What this approach does is challenge the way these problems have been seen to be *the fault of those struggling to manage their eating*. It is the blaming and shaming that are wrong – because these just make us feel bad and do not encourage or inspire us to try harder if we need to. An accusatory approach based on blaming and shaming does not offer solutions and often makes it even less likely we will lose weight for the sake of our health.

## Jane's story

We can get more insight into how complex these difficulties can be, and how mixed messages can make us feel ashamed and self-critical, by looking at one individual's experience. Jane's story is typical of many people who have attempted to diet. It shows how something as supposedly easy as losing weight can be a very complicated and tricky business, and how this struggle can often be linked with other feelings we have about ourselves.

Jane was in the healthy weight range for her height. However, she always had felt very dissatisfied with her body. While she was growing up, she was a little overweight for her height and was often teased by her peers about her appearance. She learned to think about her body all the time, because that was the aspect of her that attracted criticism, and also to be fearful of what people thought about her. She believed that she would never meet people who would accept her as she was. She believed that the only way she could be accepted by others was to be thinner; and so, ever since her early teens she has been on and off diets.

In some ways, Jane was a relatively successful dieter. Although her weight fluctuated in a range of about two stone, she was able to keep it within the healthy weight range. However, she believed she needed to be constantly vigilant about what she ate and when she ate. She had lots of rules about this, and did her best to avoid eating socially so that people could not pressure her into eating things she thought she should not eat.

Like many dieters, Jane often found that she could not keep to her strict rules about eating for more than two or three months. When she gained weight after a diet (as most dieters will) she became very afraid, and after a week or two she would try to diet again. Jane felt that the best way to keep her desire for her 'forbidden foods' and her hunger in check was to constantly call herself names – names like 'fatty', 'pig' and 'fat cow', some of which she had learned from the children who had bullied and teased her when she was young, and some of which she had made up herself. Not surprisingly, Jane felt low and miserable when she called herself these names. Because Jane was fearful of her weight, because it was associated in her mind with social unacceptability and shame, when she felt over-weight those feelings of being pointed at and ashamed would come back to her. Those feelings would then trigger a sinking feeling and a sense of frustration, which quickly turned into self-criticism: 'What's the matter with me? Why can't I keep to my diets?' Out of this would come feelings of anger and contempt and more name-calling.

Sometimes, when she felt low, Jane would stand in front of the mirror looking at bits of her body that she particularly didn't like, then calling herself even more names. At other times she would scream and shout at herself as she tried on clothes (usually the ones she could only fit in at her lowest weight), or look at pictures of herself in the past and predict future misery if she did not lose weight. Sometimes Jane could not stand the misery that dieting caused her and would have what she called a 'stuff it' moment, when she would give up dieting and eat a lot of her 'forbidden foods'. At these times food would sometimes give her comfort and relief, but also was a way of punishing herself.

Jane's rejection of dieting showed a more rebellious side of her that was struggling to feel free – and in some ways was vital to her moving forward. However, as you can imagine, she had a real battle going on inside herself, between the angry, 'stuff it' part of her and the fear-driven part that wanted to control her eating. If we are honest, we can all feel that battle in ourselves sometimes – between the angry, 'stuff it', 'what the hell, let's just party' side and the anxious, 'keep control' side.

So Jane had two problems. One was linked to her eating and weight, and the other, more serious, was about her relationship with herself – which was negative, attacking and rejecting. Self-criticism of this type never creates confidence, encouragement, enthusiasm, sustained effort or genu-ine efforts to take responsibility. At best it can create a temporary, fearful falling into line, which is what it did for Jane.

When I met Jane, it became clear that her relationship with food and eating had little to do with managing her physical health. Rather, it was tied up with managing her painful memories from the past and her fear of bullying and rejection. Given how horrible these events made her school years, it is understandable that Jane would try to manage her size and shape to avoid further rejection as an adult. But one of the unintended consequences of doing so was that she became a bully to herself, and, instead of finding new ways to manage relationships and seeking out people who would support her rather than criticize her, she got caught up in a vicious circle of dieting, self-attack, low mood and binge-eating. This in turn left her feeling even more fearful of rejection by other people and led to her weight yo-yoing by about two stone, even though she remained in a 'healthy' weight range.

These unintended consequences of trying to manage our 'see-food-and-eat-it' brain and our body's size and shape can frequently lead to our feeling more distressed, and even to more weight gain (as we will see in Chapter 3).

It is for people like Jane – like most of us, including me – that this book is written. Jane was able to use many of the skills we will explore later to help her end this vicious cycle and develop a more compassionate relationship with her eating and her body.

## Food, eating and the need for self-compassion

Here in the West we live in a culture that dictates what our body size should be and links this image with success in our relationships and in our professional lives, and with our self-esteem. And yet I have never met anyone, in either my professional or my personal life (and that includes me) who is completely happy with their body size and shape. Indeed, all of us can find fault with parts of our bodies if we look hard enough. If you don't believe this, imagine standing right in front of a mirror and looking closely at a part of your body you feel happy with, trying to spot small flaws and imperfections you may not have noticed before. If you tell yourself that these things are important and will have a bearing on how other people see you or treat you, you will find an easy path to dissatisfaction with your body. In fact, when people are anxious about their looks that's exactly what they sometimes do – stare into the mirror looking for flaws and things they are dissatisfied with. This is not a good idea, really. When we focus in like this, our brain can easily give us a feeling of dissatisfaction, even with things we were satisfied with before!

On the other hand, we know that the numbers of people who are very overweight – that is, clinically obese, which is defined as having a BMI of 35 or over, or morbidly obese (having a BMI over 40) are rising sharply. Recent estimates suggest that over 25 per cent of adults in the UK are now clinically obese; this is almost double the rate of ten years ago. In the United States of America 31 per cent of adults are estimated to have a BMI over 30. And the picture is even worse for our children, whose overall levels of obesity and rates of increase are higher than their parents'.

As we have already seen, there is a range of reasons why obesity has become such a serious problem, including changes to our diet, the increasing availability of food, advertising, our changing lifestyles and the reduction in physical activity and exercise. It's very clear that the *cause* of the problem lies not in individuals but in our societies. You might think, then, that it would be best tackled by trying to develop social interventions that target the food industry and increase activity levels. In fact, quite the opposite has happened, with yet another industry growing up – the diet industry.

Most of the diets marketed by this new industry tell us that significant reductions in energy intake and increases in energy output through exercise will give us complete control over our size and shape. There is also the suggestion that weight loss is both desirable and sustainable for everyone. Anyone who has been on a diet, or seen their friends and family dieting, will probably know that things are not as straightforward as this. Indeed, the evidence suggests that most diets, and particularly those involving severe or rapid weight loss, are likely to end in failure and in all probability further weight gain. Furthermore, dieting can have significant physical and psychological consequences, particularly if your weight goes up and down repeatedly – called 'yo-yo' dieting – or you lose weight too rapidly. There is also the psychological harm that can arise if we keep trying and failing at things, which doesn't exactly inspire confidence in ourselves or build self-esteem – and yet this is the common experience of dieters.

We need to recognize that, for health reasons, it's important that we eat enough healthy food, maintain a relatively stable and healthy body weight, and provide our body with the degree of both physical activity and rest that it needs. We also need to recognize that we need to take responsibility, as best we can, for doing all these things, but that we are living in a society that doesn't really help us to do any of them. So we have to find a way of helping ourselves; and, as we will see in the rest of this book, this means learning to be deeply compassionate to ourselves in tackling these difficulties so that we can feel encouraged and supported, are able to fail without feeling ashamed or critical, and can just pick ourselves up and keep going.

## What is a 'healthy body weight'?

Let's now look more deeply into the health aspects of weight. Medical professionals today calculate a 'healthy body weight' using something called the 'body mass index' or BMI, which I've already referred to. It's not hard to work out your own BMI. First multiply your height in metres by itself. Then divide your weight in kilograms by this number – and the number you end up with is your BMI. (You might want to look at www.eatwell.gov.uk/healthydiet/healthyweight/bmicalculator/ to help you calculate your BMI.)

For example, Jane weighs 70 kilograms (11 stone) and is 1.7 metres (5 feet 7 inches) tall. So to work out her BMI she would first multiply 1.7 by 1.7, giving a figure of 2.89, and then divide 70 by 2.89. This gives her BMI, which is just over 24.

People with a BMI in the range 20–25 are believed to have a healthy body weight. So Jane could weigh anything between 58 kg (9 st. 2 lb) and 75 kg (11 st. 10 lb) – a range of 17 kg, or 2 st. 6 lb – and still be at a healthy weight for her height.

This BMI range, which gives people considerable scope in what their healthy weight can be, represents a move away from the old-fashioned (and unsustainable) very narrow 'ideal weight' bands, which were mainly based upon the dictates of fashion rather than health.

Many health professionals believe that risks to our health increase significantly if we have a BMI of over 30 or below 18. However, even this wider band – at the upper end, at least – has been questioned by some health professionals. There is now good evidence to suggest that some people with a BMI of over 30 may face significantly fewer health risks than people who are in the 'healthy' weight range, if they are physically active and eat healthily according to their bodies' needs.

There are many myths around healthy body weight. As we've already seen, obesity is rising in many Western countries, and very substantial excess weight – described by medical professionals as 'morbid obesity' – does pose risks to health. However, there are other statistics to be taken into account. We are collectively a bit heavier (about 6–11 lb) than the previous generation; but we are also taller (by about 1 inch on average), and are likely to live up to seven years longer.

So there's no need to panic! The key issue for our own well-being is not to let collective changes blind us to our own individual needs, or automatically to assume that we need to lose weight. We may live in a culture where being a little taller and a little heavier than our parents is actually more likely to mean we are healthy – *if* we also eat what our body needs and are physically active. However, if we overeat a lot – especially if we eat a lot of foods that are not particularly good for us – and are much heavier than we would be if we ate what our body needed, then it can only be a good thing to address this in a compassionate manner to improve our health and sense of well-being.

So we know, then, that our bodies can be healthy in a relatively wide weight range. When we are at a healthy body weight, we can function to the best of our abilities, physically, intellectually and emotionally. It's important to realize that (apart from greatly excess levels, as I've already said) it's often not weight *itself* that poses risks to our health so much as *not caring for* our bodies by providing them with consistent levels of adequate nutrition and activity. Attempts to achieve rapid weight loss, often driven by dissatisfaction with our body shape or as a way of helping us feel in control of difficult emotions, are no more likely to improve our health than rapid or prolonged weight gain. Weight does play a role in our health, but as one of a wide range of other factors.

## How our bodies regulate their own weight: the 'set-point system'

Our bodies have evolved to maintain a set weight, which is determined by factors such as genetics and the level of nutrition received in the womb or as a child. People who do not diet or overeat very much tend to maintain a relatively stable weight throughout their adult lives. When weight changes do occur, biological mechanisms (e.g. increases/decreases in appetite, changes in body metabolism) then act to restore weight to a stable level. This 'set-point' system evolved to maintain our body weight at a level that is healthy for each of us. It is possible to override our 'set point', but it takes a great deal of effort to keep our weight below our set point in the in the long term, and doing so poses a significant risk to our health. Our bodies find it easier to maintain our weight above our set point, but again this can also affect our health.

In animals and young children the 'set point' is relatively easily maintained by the hunger–satiety system – in plain English, whether we feel empty or full! As we grow up our relationship with food becomes far more complex and we can choose to ignore our hunger–satiety system, for example by not eating when we are hungry or eating when we feel full. Our bodies are able to cope with day-to-day fluctuations in eating (for example, overdoing it at Christmas) and will normally restore our body weight by short-term changes in our appetite and metabolic rate. However, our bodies have not evolved to cope with prolonged periods of starvation, overeating or irregular eating patterns. These can override our body's natural ability to stabilize our weight. Our bodies also work on a 'better safe than sorry' principle, which evolved in times when famine was a constant threat. So if we do lose a significant amount of weight and then go back to eating normally again, our set point goes up to allow us to gain more weight in defence against future 'famine'. This is why, on average, a person who goes on a diet ends up in the long term 3 lb heavier than they were before they began the diet.

The 'set-point' system is a complex one. Our body regulates our weight and eating through two main mechanisms: the rate at which our body naturally uses up energy (the metabolic rate), and our experiences of feeling hungry or having had enough food (the hunger–satiety system). In addition, there are several ways in which the natural 'set-point' mechanism can be overridden: some of them involve deliberate attempts to manage our weight or feelings, while others happen without any direct intention on our part. These are shown in Figure 2.1.

## Overeating, the set point and the hunger–satiety system

In the previous section we looked at how our bodies can cope with temporary, short-term changes in our eating patterns. However, most people who overeat in the long term will deliberately or accidentally override their hunger–satiety system and thus change their natural set point – their natural, individual healthy body weight. In this chapter we

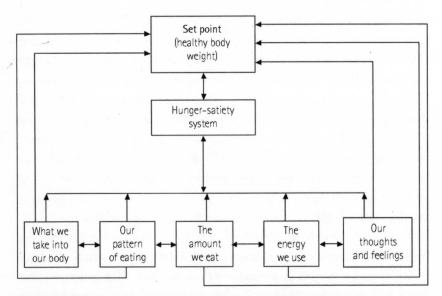

**Figure 2.1:** Ways we can override the hunger–satiety system

will explore how this can happen via the body's natural response to things we take into it, our eating patterns, and the amount of energy we eat and use up (the first four boxes in the bottom row of Figure 2.1). In Chapter 3 we will explore the complex relationship between our social relationships, emotions and eating (the last box in the figure). We will see in particular how central self-criticism is to many people's attempts to manage their eating – even, in some cases, turning into self-disgust and self-loathing.

Clearly you may not do all of the things listed below. However, it is useful to explore the things you *do* do, deliberately or accidentally, that influence your body's natural tendency to keep you at your own healthy weight. Again, it is important to remember that you are not to blame for the side-effects of doing these things. Many of the things you have been doing that work to override your body's set point are likely to have come from a genuine attempt to improve your physical or psychological health. The diet industry is powerful and well established, whereas much of the information you need to understand the unintended consequences of managing your weight is not yet generally available; so it's all too easy to set out with the best of intentions without realizing that some of what you are doing may actually be hindering rather than helping you.

As a result of – probably unwittingly – altering the balance of your hunger–satiety system, it's quite probably that you will be out of touch with, or afraid of, your body's natural response to hunger or to being overfed. This section is designed to help you understand this system and to begin to work with it, rather than against it, as you develop a more healthy relationship with eating.

## What we take into our bodies

### *Fluid*

Besides air, food is the third most important thing that we take into our body; the second most important is, of course, fluid. How much we drink can have a significant effect on our eating and our health. Many weight-loss diets advise people to drink a glass or more of water before or during eating so they will feel full, and hence eat less.

Given how important fluid is to us, it is not surprising that we have evolved powerful mechanisms for dealing with fluid intake, just as we have for hunger. However, just as in hunger, this mechanism can be pretty complex. If we eat less we also tend to drink less, and the more we eat the more we need to drink. So drinking a lot of water when we are eating less (as many diets suggest) can upset this mechanism. Training our bodies to drink water rather than eat when we are hungry will leave us feeling full, even bloated, but can also make it very difficult for us to know when we have had too much (or too little) food. If we drink a great deal too much, particularly without eating, this can lead to imbalances in the body that can seriously affect our health, and in the most extreme cases can kill us.

Over 70 per cent of our weight is made up of fluid. Rapid weight loss is often seen as desirable in diet programmes, but this usually relies on dehydration and so is not sustainable in the long term: as soon as we put fluid back into our body, the weight tends to go back on, and even increase for a while. What happens when we lose weight rapidly, through dieting or a lot of activity, is that we lose water and glycogen. Glycogen is starch, and we store 1–3 lb of it in our liver and muscles. It is the body's equivalent of rocket fuel, an easily accessible source of energy. Understandably, the body does not like running out of this handy resource, and if it runs low, we are evolved to snatch it back as soon as some carbohydrate is eaten. Glycogen needs to be stored in solution, and we need 1–3 lb of water to store 1 lb of glycogen. So if you use up 1 lb of glycogen you will actually lose 2–4 lb total weight. Conversely, if you put back 1lb of glycogen, you will gain 2–4 lb total weight.

Suppose, for example, that you go on a strict diet for a week before your holiday, eating very little, and also exercise hard – perhaps going to the gym, and for a run, every day. Perhaps by the end of the week the scales tell you that you've lost 8 lb. You're delighted – now you can feel better on the beach. On holiday you eat normally – not excessively – and do a fair bit of walking and swimming, but nothing very energetic. You get home and stand on the scales and are horrified to discover that not only have you put that 8 lb back on, you've put on another 2 lb as well! All that has happened in fact is that you lost 2 lb of glycogen in that week of near-starvation, which took another 6 lb of water with it. This sudden depletion of your glycogen stores rang warning bells in your body, so as soon as you started eating some carbohydrates again on holiday it made sure to get back all the glycogen it could, replacing a bit more than the 2 lb you lost so that, with the extra water needed to store it, you gained a little more weight than you'd lost in the first place. Not very encouraging, is it?

## Alcohol and other drugs

It's all too easy to think that weight is all about food, and in fact we are often unaware of the effects that other things we put in our bodies can have on our eating and weight. It is not surprising, given the prejudice and stigma attached to being even a little overweight, that some people are so desperate to change that they will deliberately take legal and illegal drugs in their attempts to lose weight: These include:

- laxatives

- diuretics (e.g. caffeine)

- amphetamines

- diet pills

- thyroxin

- insulin (necessary for diabetics, but sometimes misused)

- cigarettes.

It is important to acknowledge that these do work, at least in the short term, for some people. Some of these drugs (such as diet pills) will affect appetite directly; others (such as cigarettes) are likely to be used as a food substitute, or a substitute for emotional eating. All carry health risks – for example, smoking is linked to cancer, and caffeine to disturbed sleep – and most people are likely to gain weight when they stop using them. Some, such as diuretics (including caffeine) and laxatives, give the illusion of weight loss:

but, as we have seen in talking about glycogen, this is usually by causing rapid fluctuations in fluid content that are not translated into long-term weight loss.

So while taking any of these drugs can often give one a sense of control over weight gain, it is likely that this will be at best short-lived. It may actually make things worse as we give ourselves permission to overeat because we will later be taking something to get rid of the food (such as a laxative).

Other people may deliberately or accidentally stimulate their hunger by taking:

- alcohol

- antihistamines

- steroids

- some anti-depressant or anti-psychotic medication

- marijuana.

These are substances that people often take to manage difficult feelings, without recognizing the longer-term effects they are likely to have on our mood, appetite or ability to manage our eating. Some people, of course, have no choice but to take medication to manage medical or psychiatric conditions; however, they are often not aware of the side-effects this will have for their weight.

Perhaps the most interesting, and certainly the most widely used, of these substances is alcohol. Most of us know that alcohol contains a lot of calories, and that it reduces our inhibitions – including those about eating. More importantly for those of us trying to manage our eating, it also stimulates appetite in the short term (how else could I explain the desperate need for a kebab at 2 a.m.?). Although in the short term alcohol can feel as if it relaxes us and helps us feel good, it can actually have a negative effect on our mood, leaving us wanting another drink when we come home at the end of the hectic evening. So we have that extra glass of wine, which reduces our inhibitions more, which in turn reduces our ability to eat sensibly – and we raid the fridge for snacks. Then in the morning we can feel a bit annoyed with ourselves again. This is a very common cycle – and most of us never stop to ask ourselves whether maybe the lifestyles we're leading that send us to alcohol for relaxation are just too stressful.

So the role alcohol plays in our weight is complex. It is linked to the amount we drink and its effect on our moods, our appetites, and our ability to resist our desires.

## Our pattern of eating

Our eating patterns can have a profound effect on our body's natural mechanism for regulating our weight. We live in a world that all too often makes extreme and conflicting demands on us. On the one hand, often it is difficult to respond to our natural urges to eat regularly, for example because we work in jobs that do not allow us time to take proper breaks to look after our bodies, or because we are running around looking after a house and children and rarely have time for a proper meal. On the other hand, our culture promotes the belief that exercising extreme control over our eating habits is the only way to manage our weight – or even to be happy!

There are three major eating patterns that people who overeat tend to fall into:

- the starve–eat cycle
- the starve–binge–purge cycle
- chaotic eating.

### The starve-eat cycle

Many people will at some time deliberately attempt to lose weight, either by restricting eating or exercising more or both. As a result 'biological starvation' takes place: this is when our body is using up more energy than it is consuming. The body's natural response to biological starvation is to make us want to eat. This was the pattern we evolved to help us deal with times of famine, to encourage us to go looking for more food.

We learned a lot about what happens to the human body when it is deprived of adequate nutrition in the late 1940s and 1950s, when psychologists and doctors tried to work out how to safely re-feed famine and concentration camp victims after the end of the Second World War. In a pioneering study, Ansel Keys and his colleagues in America found that even at the calorie levels suggested by most diet programmes, their volunteers experienced profound psychological and physical side-effects. These included:

- preoccupation with food and eating

- episodes of overeating

- low mood and irritability

- becoming obsessional

- difficulty in concentrating

- loss of interest in everyday activities

- loss of sexual desire

- feeling unsociable

- relationship difficulties.

The starvation response appears to follow a specific pattern that is not confined to humans but can be found across species. It has two distinct phases: initially the body drives us to find food, and then, if these attempts fail, the body helps us to conserve its energy stores. The side-effects of these responses can reinforce our attempts to lose weight, particularly in the early stages of a diet. However, the effects in phase two can often lead to weight gain, and in turn to fear of our appetite and desire for food. It's worth going into a bit of detail here about how the starvation response works in someone who goes on a diet, because it is very important to understand this if we are to understand why attempts to manage our weight so often founder. I'm describing the most extreme forms of the various features, but everyone who diets will experience them to some degree.

## Phase 1: The initial search for food

Weight loss is relatively easy in the early weeks of dieting, mainly because – as we saw earlier in this section when thinking about fluid intake – we lose fluid and glycogen first. This can help motivate us further to continue with our diet.

In these first weeks we get an initial burst of energy and tend to feel in a good mood (a 'starvation high'). This response evolved to help us get up and look for food. So if we are dieting we learn (at least in the early stages) that eating less makes us feel better. We learn to associate not eating with feeling good.

So far – it seems – so good. But the next feature of this phase often causes problems if we're dieting. Food becomes more important than anything else. We become preoccupied with thoughts of food and eating, and more sensitized to food smells or taste. So if we are dieting we will often be more tempted by foods than usual. If we 'give in' to this temptation and eat them, we often (wrongly) see this as a lack of willpower, and this is one of the points where we can become very self-critical of our 'weakness'.

Another effect in this phase is that we become more emotionally detached – that is, our feelings become somewhat blunted – because when we were really starving we could not afford to let any emotional distractions get in the way of our search for food and survival. Again, if we're dieting it seems to us that losing weight actually does help us manage our emotions.

We also find it more difficult to sleep and may become more restless, because we cannot afford to rest when we need to look for food to survive. Problems with sleep are common in people who diet, and sleep deprivation in turn has a profound effect on our appetite. When we are tired, we tend to produce more of the hormones that make us feel hungry: we feel less full and our appetite increases. We also become depressed and irritable. None of this is good news for those of us who are anxious about eating more, or who tend to eat to manage our feelings.

As we lose weight our body adjusts our metabolic rate downwards to conserve energy, so it becomes harder to lose more weight (this is what dieters call a 'plateau'). This phase is often very frustrating for those of us wanting to lose weight; it often drives us to even more extreme attempts at weight loss or into the starve–binge–purge pattern we will look at next.

## Phase 2: Losing the hunt for food

Again I have outlined the more extreme forms of the various aspects of this phase, as they would have occurred in our hunter-gatherer ancestors in times of real famine; but again, everyone who diets will experience them to some degree.

As we lose more weight and cannot find food, the body starts to take emergency steps to preserve energy:

- It stops pumping blood to our fingers and toes to reduce heat loss.

- It slows down the rate at which we empty our stomach, leading to problems of constipation and bloating (so we feel very full).

- We are even less able to concentrate.

- We feel exhausted. By this point our rate of weight loss has slowed down even more: we have given up the hunt for food and our only hope is to stop moving and survive until someone brings it to us.

- We experience mood swings, feeling increasingly detached from everyday living, and tend to isolate ourselves from others. This may be an evolved response to save us from the distress of our imminent death and allow our families to leave us and carry on the hunt for food.

- Eventually our body begins literally to eat itself to survive: it gets vitamins and minerals from our bones (giving us osteoporosis), and starts to draw on our vital organs and muscles to provide calories.

- Finally, if there is still no food coming in, we die.

Of course, most of us who diet will not get to the last stage of this sequence! But there is good evidence to suggest that those who lose weight by deliberately giving the body less than it needs, or to keep their body below its set point, for long periods of time will experience problems with their physical and psychological health. Fortunately, as we will see in later chapters, managing your weight doesn't have to be a constant battle with your own survival instincts: the good news is that the body has very good ways of judging how much it needs to eat, and if we trust it and learn to listen to it rather than feeling we have to fight our impulses, our physical and psychological health will benefit as a result.

## The eating response to starvation

Just as our bodies have evolved a fixed set of responses to the absence of food, so they have also evolved very efficient survival mechanisms to make the most of food when it becomes available again. These affect:

- what food we eat

- how fast we eat

- how our weight changes

Our initial response to starvation is to try to eat – anything! This includes things we would not normally contemplate. This can break down the cultural or food preference barriers to eating we may have. At the most extreme, this can mean eating things that are otherwise taboo for religious or cultural reasons (including animals or even other humans). In less extreme circumstances, for example, if we're on a diet, it can mean eating things we really don't like: how many of us have found ourselves, late at night in the kitchen, hoovering up unappetizing leftovers or eating cold baked beans from the tin? Yes, I thought it wasn't just me!

As most dieters have a lot of rules in place about what they can and can't eat, this drive to eat can cause real difficulties. We can become very self-critical when we break our rules, seeing ourselves as weak or inadequate in some way when all we're doing is responding to our body's natural need to recover from a famine – even if it's one we have imposed on ourselves.

Also, once food is available again we usually eat more and faster than we would normally. In evolutionary terms this makes sense if we do not know where our next meal is coming from! For a dieter it seems that a week's 'success' can be wiped out in ten minutes.

As we have been eating less, our body has already slowed our metabolic rate down to conserve energy; this means that, when we start eating again, our weight tends to rise relatively rapidly, and at first it will stabilize at a higher weight than before the 'famine' began. This is the 'better safe than sorry' principle in action, giving us some extra energy stores, particularly in the form of fat, in case famine returns. This can be very disappointing if we have deliberately tried to lose weight: extra weight gain is seen as a sign of failure, and often sparks off another spate of dieting. Many serial dieters will recognize this repeated cycle of weight loss followed by weight gain. In fact if you want to gain weight the best way to do it is to diet!

Now for the good news. Our body does not continually gain weight if food supplies are enough for our needs. Gradually our metabolic rate and eating returns to normal, and as excess energy stores are no longer necessary, we gradually lose weight to our pre-diet level – but *only if we don't diet again*. However strange this may sound to habitual dieters, if the food supply continues to be adequate, and our activity levels don't exceed our need for food, then gradually eating and weight return to normal.

## The starve–binge–purge cycle

When we go without food for more than three or four hours it becomes increasingly difficult to ignore our body's drive to find and eat food in order to survive. After this time our blood sugar falls and we produce hormones that stimulate our appetite. If we eat, particularly if we eat foods with some fat in them, this will turn off these hormones and trigger other hormonal changes that give us feelings of fullness, so we stop eating. We have already explored the various ways we can override this system, particularly by dieting. If we were in a genuine famine, our body's drive to find food would mean that when we came across any we would eat as much as possible in order to replenish our energy supplies, because of our uncertainty about when we would next be able to eat.

Eating larger amounts of food than is normal in an uncontrolled fashion is referred to as 'binge-eating' or 'bingeing'. However, whereas primitive men and women at the end of a famine would relax and tuck in, finding the presence of food a reason for rejoicing, people who are deliberately trying to lose weight or control their food intake tend to find bingeing a very upsetting experience. They often do not understand or are scared of their body's attempts to push them back to a healthy weight and an adequate intake of food. They tend to experience feelings of fear (of weight gain and of loss of control), guilt, shame and panic about wanting/needing to eat.

These feelings can then lead them to the 'purge' stage of the cycle to get rid of the food they have eaten. Purging includes any method of getting rid of calories or food itself (e.g. excessive exercise, vomiting or use of laxatives). As well as having dangerous physiological effects for the body, these reactions also make the body feel it is being starved even more. Most people who diet will recognize this cycle, even if only in a mild form that sends them off to the gym for an hour after eating half a packet of biscuits. In its most extreme form it is the pattern associated with the eating disorder bulimia nervosa. However, most dieters are more likely to follow episodes of bingeing with further episodes of dieting. This pattern tends to lead to weight gain, mainly because of the effects of dieting on our metabolic rate that we looked at earlier.

So you can see how this pattern can become a vicious circle of dieting, bingeing and purging, which is emotionally very difficult to manage and can have very serious health consequences. Figure 2.2 shows how this cycle fits together.

## Chaotic eating

Now of course, most of us, when we are trying to do something about our weight, do not fall neatly into the mild versions of the starve–eat or

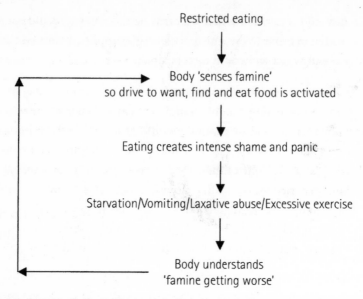

**Figure 2.2:** The starve–binge–purge cycle

*Source*: Adapted from C. G. Fairburn and P. Cooper, 'Eating disorders', in K. Hawton, P. M. Salkovskis, J. Kirk and D.M. Clark (eds), *Cognitive Behaviour Therapy for Psychiatric Problems: A Practical Guide* (Oxford: Oxford University Press, 1989).

starve–binge–purge cycles. Some of us may fluctuate between the two. Some people find that even *thinking* about beginning a diet can trigger an eating response. This may be particularly true for 'serial dieters'. Many of us find that our eating just becomes chaotic, veering between episodes of dieting and episodes of overeating, both to varying degrees, so that we lose any sense of what it is to eat 'normally'. The important thing for us to remember is that if we eat chaotically our body will tend to be on higher alert for signs of famine and so is likely to trigger the hunger response more readily.

It is possible for our body to respond to our need to eat even if we try to stop eating. For example, some people develop what is called 'night eating disorder'. This is a form of sleepwalking where individuals may not be aware of what they are eating because they do it while they are asleep. Others may develop a bingeing pattern but cannot or do not attempt to compensate for their binges by purging or restricting their food intake, and so may put on weight. This weight gain leads to an increase in their metabolic rate. So, to maintain their weight at the new level they will initially feel hungrier than before or feel hungry even when they are full. This may mean they eat more in the long term, possibly leading to further gradual weight gain.

Some dieters can keep to their strict rules most of the time, but when they break them have the 'stuff it' response. They get angry with themselves for breaking their diet, and decide that if they have broken a rule they might as well break it properly! This can lead to binge-eating. Yet others may use food to punish themselves for being unable to keep to their diet.

It is important to realize that these patterns are followed the world over by people who diet. If you recognize any of them in your own life, remember: they are just a normal human response to trying to diet and lose weight. If you think about the number of rules you have to keep to when you are on a diet, you'll see that it is impossible to keep them all, even if other people don't tempt you to break them: your natural need to eat means that you will break them. If you criticize yourself, or see your desire to eat as a sign of personal weakness, this may motivate you to start dieting again – but it is also likely to lead to a lifetime struggling with your weight, eating and mood.

## The energy we use

Having looked at the intake side of the equation, let's now look at the output side. All the energy we get comes from food, and we use it in three ways:

- to keep our body ticking over – for example, to keep our hearts beating, our blood going round, and all our other vital organs functioning;

- to digest the food we eat;

- to fuel whatever activity we do.

If we eat just the amount of food we need for these three things, we are in 'energy balance'. That is, 'energy in' equals 'energy out': we do not store energy, nor are we deprived of it, and our weight remains stable. If we eat more energy than we use, it is stored as fat to be used at a later date. If we eat less energy than we use, our body interprets this as biological starvation and responds in the ways we saw in the previous section.

## Ticking over

The largest portion of the energy we use up every day (between 60 and 75 per cent) is used just to keep our bodies functioning. The energy we eat is measured in calories, and as a rule of thumb most adults need about 1,400 calories per day just to 'tick over'. This would keep us alive if all we did was to lie completely still all day. The rate at which we use energy (without doing anything other than lying still) is called our 'resting metabolic rate' (RMR). Our RMR increases when we eat more, and decreases when we eat less than we need, as the body tries to conserve its dwindling energy stocks. There are also small differences between individuals in metabolic rates: for example, people with a higher proportion of muscle and bone, compared to fat, tend to have a higher metabolic rate, and our metabolic rate needs to reduce a little as we get older. But the requirement for about 1,400 calories a day just to keep ticking over is a pretty good rule of thumb.

## Digestion

Eating and digesting food actually use energy – but not much: on average, around 150 calories a day! So, to cover our RMR and the 'cost' in energy of taking in energy, we need to consume something like 1,550 calories a day.

## Physical activity

Of course, none of us actually lies still all day, every day – so to get at the total number of calories we use, we have to add those we need to maintain our RMR, those we use up eating and digesting, and the calories we need to fuel whatever physical activity we do. This includes all the ordinary things like walking to the bathroom in the morning and moving paper across the desk as well as 'taking exercise' like playing football or going to the gym. Most people who are neither very inactive nor extremely active will use something between 2,000 and 2,500 calories per day.

This third area of energy use, physical activity, is the most variable. For example, someone who does no physical activity (i.e. sits around all day) may need to add just 100 calories to the 1,550 they need for their body to tick over and to feed itself; whereas someone who is very active may need to add 3,000 calories a day to the same basic 1,550.

Interestingly, just as the body responds to our eating too little by slowing down energy use, if we eat too much it responds by trying to use up more. There is wide variation in how well our bodies do this, but everyone tends to increase their physical activity when they eat more. Scientists have proven what I call the 'Boxing Day Effect' – the overwhelming desire to go for a walk after eating too much on Christmas Day! They found that humans naturally increase their physical activity after being forced to eat more than their body needs. Much of this activity appeared to be involuntary (i.e. fidgeting). If we tune into this mechanism then, even if we do overeat, it is unlikely that we will gain weight.

Much of the information put out by the diet industry does not focus on the significant effects exercise can have on metabolic rate and health, implying that restricting eating, particularly by following low-calorie diets, will do the trick. In fact, as we have already seen, because our bodies have well-established mechanisms designed to keep us healthy, the most likely outcome of severely restricting what we eat is that our metabolic rate will slow down. On the other hand, even moderately increasing physical activity has a beneficial effect on both our physical and our psychological health. It works with our bodies by helping them to increase their metabolic rate, which in turn will help us to avoid gaining weight – as long as we put in enough calories to stop our body going into a starvation state.

## Excessive exercise and activity

As I have just said, regular enjoyable exercise and activity can improve our physical and mental health. However, some people use exercise not only as a way of keeping fit and relaxed but as a way to try to reduce their weight below its natural set point, to alter their natural shape and/or to manage difficult feelings. I am not suggesting exercise and physical activity are bad things – far from it! However, if we are to develop a compassionate approach to our bodies, it is important to recognize the potentially damaging effects that *too much* exercise can have on our health. For example:

- If no additional calories are taken in to compensate for those used in excessive exercise our body will read this sustained energy loss as 'famine', and this can trigger the starve–eat cycle or the starve–binge–purge cycle.

- Excessive exercise can do physical damage, for example to joints and muscles.

- If exercise becomes an obsession, this can do psychological damage: for example, we may start to get depressed, agitated, angry or anxious if we are unable to exercise as much as we want to.

- Obsessive exercise can also damage our social, personal and working lives if we get to the point of putting it ahead of other areas of life.

If you're not sure whether you might be exercising excessively, a good way to approach the question is to ask yourself if you treat your body like a professional athlete would. They have planned rest days, will not exercise if they are ill or injured, maintain adequate levels of food intake, and tend to enjoy what their body can do for them!

### SUMMARY

We humans have evolved a complex system to help us manage our eating in times of famine and make the most of food when the famine passes. This system is sensitive to a whole range of deliberate or accidental changes in our eating and appetite. Sometimes we can become afraid of, or even blame ourselves for, our body's natural attempts to stabilize our weight at a level that is healthy for us. Learning to take a compassion focused approach to this area of our lives will involve coming to understand more about the ways in which we have affected our 'set-point' weight and getting back in touch with our body's natural systems for managing our weight and eating. Many people find this very difficult, particularly as it involves ignoring the advice that many in the diet industry (and many health professionals) give and the hope that it offers – that, if only we could keep to a low-calorie diet, we could all be as thin was we want, and that this is the path to happiness!

In the next chapter we will explore how our feelings can influence our eating, and how we can learn different ways to deal with some difficult emotions.

# 3 Making sense of overeating, part 2: eating and our feelings

In Chapter 2 we explored the ways in which we can deliberately or accidentally interfere with our body's natural ways of keeping us healthy and managing our urges to overeat. Perhaps the most powerful way in which we override these natural mechanisms is in eating as a response to factors in our social environment and to our emotional states.

Now, emotions are tricky things. Our basic emotions – our capacity to feel anger, anxiety, sadness, joy and lust – are older than our human species, having evolved many millions of years ago. They can be easily activated and can be powerful, because the feelings we identify as emotions are accompanied by the surge through our bodies of chemicals called hormones. This means that when we feel strong emotions they arouse in us desires and urges to act – to fight, to run away, to cry or to celebrate. Sometimes, if we have not learned to recognize, understand or cope with our emotions, they can seem overwhelming. Sometimes we can worry that if we don't control them we will simply fall apart.

Also, of course, we can have a conflict of emotions. For example, we can be very angry with somebody whom we love, so because we don't want to hurt them, we don't say anything but still feel resentful; or we can be very angry with somebody whom we're frightened of, so again we don't say anything, but later become angry and berate ourselves: 'Why don't I stand up for myself?' we ask. We can be criticized for being too emotional or not emotional enough. Often our feelings (or at least showing them) can be seen as a sign of weakness or a source of fear or shame. So we can feel ashamed of our feelings. Interestingly, there seem to be different rules about feelings and how to handle them for different genders and different cultures. These messages can be quite confusing: for example, 'men don't cry' (but 'new men' should), or 'women shouldn't show anger' (but 'new' women should).

Many people use food to deal with their emotions. Sometimes as children they were given food (chocolates, sweets, cakes) when they were upset. So instead of talking about and learning to think about their feelings they've learned simply to try to turn them off by distracting themselves with food. As they grow up, getting rid of, avoiding and turning off painful feelings becomes a way of life – and not doing so, but instead starting to allow oneself to feel and think about one's emotions, can seem very frightening. So for a host of reasons we can be very confused about our feelings and how to manage them. In this chapter we will explore our emotions and how they can affect our eating.

## Learning to eat

Eating has always been a social experience for humans. It helps us to make and keep social relationships and to celebrate important events in our lives. We will begin our exploration journey by considering how feeding as an infant affects our emotions.

We know that when infants suckle this has a positive emotional impact. Infants show a typical pattern of being soothed and relaxed while feeding; but this also requires active involvement from the person doing the feeding. If baby mammals are given food, but not physical closeness, emotional warmth and eye contact, they become distressed when eating. They can even fail to grow and refuse to eat. So from a very early stage we learn to associate food and eating with emotional comfort. Indeed, some psychologists have suggested that the feeding process actually provides the beginning of social and emotional development.

We have already seen that some of our food preferences, for example our liking for sweet things, are part of our biological makeup. However, we also learn a lot about the foods we like (or dislike) and when to stop eating them as we grow up. For example, by two years of age toddlers know when they are full, but also have learned from adults what foods are supposed to be eaten for breakfast. As we grow older we learn to express certain food preferences, and will even choose what foods we will eat in different situations. Most of us will remember some foods we would eat at school, but never dream of eating at home. How we eat, too, often depends on what we learn from those around us. All too often these days meals are eaten on the go, so we have very little chance to recognize the tastes and textures of food, or the pleasure and feelings of fullness and satisfaction that taking time over eating can provide.

As we grow older we become more aware of the social nature of eating, and how it can be used to celebrate or reward, as a distraction or to soothe emotional distress. We also learn that refusing food can be very upsetting for people around us. Eating (or refusing to eat) particular types of food can become part of our religious or moral identity.

Our eating patterns, the amount we eat and our food choices change as we move from childhood into adolescence. In these years we require far more energy to fuel the changes our body will make, and around this time we also tend to become more physically active. These rapid growth spurts can leave us feeling very hungry a lot of the time; ask anyone with a teenager how often they need to refill the refrigerator! In our teens we tend to 'graze', snacking little and often. If we are left to grow through this normal stage, we will gradually learn to eat more regularly again, and are unlikely to overeat in the long run. Yet there are many social pressures, particularly on teenagers, to moderate or even limit their eating, and so many start forcing their eating into restrictive patterns, or into patterns that are fine for younger children and adults (who need less food) – for example, leaving longer gaps between meals, perhaps eating breakfast and having only a small lunch – and are discouraged from snacking. As a consequence they are actually more likely to end up overeating!

This period of growth is particularly important when we are trying to understand the link between our emotions and eating. As children faced with the physical changes that come just before and during puberty, we naturally become preoccupied with our own size and shape, and the size and shape of other people. We are also learning to deal with a rapid surge in hormones that can make us very emotional and play havoc with our sleep, and are very aware of our developing sexuality and social relationships. No wonder that our teenage years can be such a difficult time to manage. Perhaps it would have been easier if we had evolved like butterflies, whose caterpillars disappear into a chrysalis to mature and emerge a couple of months later as fully grown adults! Sadly, this isn't the case – in fact, the transition is getting longer: in Western cultures at least, puberty is beginning at a younger age, but we don't grow into our final physical state of development for at least ten years from then. This is a pretty long time; and, given the various factors that can affect our eating, it is not surprising that many of us struggle with our relationship with eating during and after adolescence.

## Understanding our emotions

All organisms have motivations to survive and reproduce. One way of thinking about emotions is that they are a way to give us signals that we are succeeding or failing in these basic tasks of life. They help us to attach meaning to events and relationships, and to recognize the things that we need. In his book *The Compassionate Mind*, Paul Gilbert outlines how we have evolved at least three types of emotional system. Each of these systems involves specific types of emotion, attention, thoughts and behaviour that can be very helpful in guiding us to meet the challenges of life.

- The first system is linked to detecting and dealing with threats, and so involves emotions like anger, anxiety and disgust.

- The second system is linked to detecting and responding to good things, such as food, friendships and sexual opportunities; it is linked to our drive to achieve and feelings of pleasure.

- The third system is associated with calm and contentment; it is linked with feelings of soothing, safety and peace, and also compassion and connection with others (affiliation).

These three systems, and their key characteristics, are shown in Figure 3.1.

### The threat system: emotions of danger and protection

We are far better at detecting and responding to unpleasant emotions than pleasant ones. This makes a lot of sense, as during the time we were evolving, like all animals, we often needed to detect threats from other

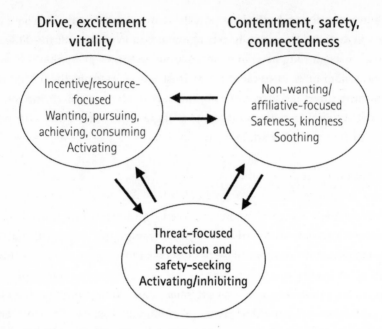

**Figure 3.1:** Three emotional regulation systems

*Source*: Adapted with permission from P. Gilbert, *The Compassionate Mind* (London: Constable & Robinson, 2009).

animals (or humans) or from our environment (such as poisonous foods). The threat system is set up to work on the 'better safe than sorry' principle. Imagine an animal, eating in a field, that suddenly hears a noise behind it. The best thing to do would be to run away, to assume that the noise came from a predator or some other threat. Nine times out of ten there will probably turn out not to have been a threat at all, but if this 'risk averse' strategy makes the animal run way the one time it needs to, it will safe its life.

So, strange as it may seem, our brains are designed to make mistakes. They are designed to attach meaning to events rapidly and to make us act quickly, because we go for 'better safe than sorry' thinking. This design also affects our memory and the things we brood on. Imagine you go shopping and nine shop assistants are very helpful but one is rude. Which one would you brood on and talk to your friends or partner about? Most likely the rude one! And we will forget the 90 per cent of shop assistants we encountered who were actually kind to us.

Another difficulty with the threat system is that it is designed to over-rule positive emotions. So, for example, imagine you're having a good time at a party when your mobile phone rings to say that your friend or child has had an accident. Or imagine that you're having a nice picnic on a sunny day in the park when you suddenly notice a swarm of bees approaching. In these situations positive emotions are quickly turned off and you turn your attention to dealing with the threat. This is why sometimes when we are stressed it's difficult to engage positive feelings: when the threat system is activated, positive emotions can be suppressed. This doesn't always happen, of course, because some kinds of threats or risks are felt to be exciting – parachute jumping, for example – but the key thing here is that we feel in control of the risk or threat, so that we notice the 'drive' (excitement) emotions more than the 'threat' emotions.

What is very interesting and relevant to us here is that some people, when they are under stress and the threat system is activated, can actually try to turn off threat emotions by activating the drive system, or with 'comfort eating'. So we can use eating as a regulator of the threat system! We will explore this in more detail in a moment.

This threat detection and protection system is associated with rapidly activated emotions such as anxiety, anger and disgust, and defensive behaviour such as the 'fight-or-flight' response, avoidance and submissiveness. It is very easy to turn on, comes with powerful emotions that are difficult to ignore and can be hard to turn down – after all, we would not want a fire bell that is hard to hear! It tends to grab our attention with both hands, and can be switched on by real events, memories and even our imagination. For example, I have a bit of a fear of heights. Even if I just close my eyes and imagine standing at the edge of a cliff and peering over, I will get feelings of vertigo and anxiety and a strong desire to think about something else!

This threat system has evolved over millions of years and operates on many levels, some of which we may not even be aware of (such as looking around the room for spiders if we are afraid of them). It is strongly influenced by our experiences, as we learn what a threat is, and what is safe in the world. It is useful in helping us detect both physical and social dangers.

Although the threat system can give us a hard time, it is important always to keep in mind that it was designed as a protection system – it is not our enemy. Once we understand it and begin to work with feelings of anxiety, anger or aloneness (or whatever feelings the threat system is 'feeding' us) we can learn to respond to it in ways that have fewer unwanted side-effects and that help us to manage life's challenges. Sadly, many of us learn quite early in life to be afraid of our threat system and the emotions it arouses – for example, to be afraid of being upset, anxious or angry. This often happens if these emotions have been responded to in a threatening way by others (for example, if we have been told off for crying, or been hit when we were angry). Even worse, we learn to experience the bodily sensations that are activated when we feel threatened (the thumping heart, the sweaty palms) as a threat in themselves if we do not understand them. We can also learn to associate other sensations (for example, hunger) or even our own body with the threat, particularly if we are worried about our eating or weight. So, as you can see, the threat system is a pretty tricky emotional system for us to manage.

## The drive system: emotions of achievement and excitement

The second important emotional system concerns emotions that give us a sense of drive, vitality and achievement. This is associated with emotions of (anticipated) pleasure and excitement. It has evolved to motivate us to do things and to actively engage in the world. We get positive feelings for doing and achieving things, such as passing an exam, going on a new date, going to a party or winning the lottery. When these things happen we become emotionally and physically activated, and often we have a desire to celebrate. When this positive feeling is interrupted or taken away – for example, when we experience setbacks or failures – we can experience this as a threat, and this in turn can motivate us to try even harder.

Let's think how this might work if we're trying to lose weight. We can often be excited by new diets and feel a great sense of achievement, even pride, when we lose a few pounds. However, after several weeks most of us will break our diet, or not lose as much weight as we did at first. This can lead to our feeling disappointed, even angry with ourselves. We can become afraid of failing, and this may make us try even harder to diet – or lead us to give up. That, in turn, as we saw with Jane in Chapter 2, can have the unintended consequence of leaving us feeling anxious, angry or even disgusted with ourselves. Clearly, no one would want to feel this way, so our fear of losing this sense of achievement can be a great motivator. Indeed, many diet programmes rely on this system and use rituals such as group weighing, with 'happy clappy' interactions to mark individual success, which are meant to give members a sense of achievement. Of course, they do not intend for those who do not lose weight to feel bad, but this tends to happen anyway! This is not to say that these groups are not helpful, but they may be helpful for different reasons – for example, because they offer affiliation with others, compassionate encouragement and support from a group. These are benefits that belong to a different emotional system, as we will now see.

## The affiliative soothing system: emotions of connection, comfort and contentment

Our third emotional system is related to soothing and contentment through our connection to others (affiliation). It is linked with the experience of peaceful well-being and feeling safe. It is also linked to being soothed. For example, imagine a parent who, seeing that their child is distressed, is loving and affectionate and hugs the child until they calm down. This very common event is actually extremely important because it tells us that humans, like other animals, can regulate their threat system and the feelings of distress and anxiety it generates by experiencing kindness, affection and compassion from others (and from ourselves). Indeed, we now know that affection and kindness are so important to humans that they actually affect how our brains develop. There are special areas of our brain and particular hormones which respond to the kindness of others, and (as recent work has shown) to self-compassion and self-kindness. So there is no doubt that kindness does help to defuse a sense of threat. Indeed, perhaps one of the greatest sources of contentment is being with people you feel loved by and under no particular pressure to achieve anything.

This type of positive emotion, that of feeling content, safe and affectionately connected to others, is a very different type of positive emotion from that gained by achievement. It can help calm down our threat detection and protection emotions and manage the unpleasant feelings we can experience if our positive feelings associated with achievement are interrupted. This system develops in childhood in response to being emotional and physically cared for, particularly when we are upset.

## Soothing and food

As we have seen, food can be a way of giving us reward or excitement, and these positive feelings can temporarily make us feel better. We can also learn to use food to soothe ourselves. Indeed, the soothing system can become very easily associated with food, particularly sweet foods, and we can learn to turn this system on by eating. This isn't surprising, given that our earliest experiences of feeding are often associated with experiences of care and affection. You can probably imagine that one of the reasons why we soothe ourselves in this way is that we can find it difficult to reach out to others and deal with our emotions in an open way (perhaps because we're ashamed of or confused by them). We might even find that we're reaching for the food before we've even realized that there is emotional distress in us. Also, if we tend to be self-critical and find it hard to be compassionate towards ourselves, then one way to tone down these negative feelings about ourselves is to turn to food.

# How are food and emotions linked?

Researchers have found that foods high in fat and sugar – the kinds of food we humans often resort to as 'comfort food' – do in fact help to reduce stress in rats. Well, of course, we are not rats; but I do know that chocolate and cake have a distinctly soothing effect on me after a hard week at work! Further research is needed to look into these effects in more detail for humans. However, it is likely that these types of food do actually operate in a way that helps us to feel soothed; they really are 'comfort food'. So part of the link between emotion and overeating may be that some foods directly help us to feel less anxious, angry, or upset.

Leaving aside the possibility of a direct chemical effect of 'comfort foods', there are several other ways we can learn to associate food and eating with our emotions. Positive emotions can become linked to food and eating via a process psychologists call 'conditioning'. This is a learning process that connects one experience with another. We all have foods that we associate with positive memories. For me it is the smell of baking, and the taste of uncooked cake mix direct from the bowl before it gets washed up. This is associated with memories of cooking with my mum and grandmother as a child. Even thinking about the smell and taste of these foods while I am writing brings back a feeling of warmth, happiness and comfort; I start to salivate and feel the urge to bake a cake!

We can also be taught by others that certain foods or tastes are associated with having a good time, or even with a certain social standing (for example, caviar), while other foods (such as chocolate) may have a more direct impact on or mood by increasing the production of chemicals in our brain that stimulate positive feelings.

We do not even have to eat the food to experience its mood-enhancing effects; for example, just imagining a nice meal, or even the smell of cooking, can lead us to feel full. We can learn to associate food as a treat, a comforter or even our friend. If it is taken away, or even if we feel we will not have it for a while, we can experience cravings.

Let's just imagine that I tell you that you must finish reading this chapter before you can go to the toilet. Do you need to pee yet? Many people tell me that just imagining this makes them want to go to the loo, even if they had no inclination before. (Don't worry, you can go to the loo now if you want to!) So thinking or being told that we are 'not allowed' to do something can produce the urge in us to do it even if we weren't thinking about it before. My clients tell me that they find this happens to them all the time around food. When they tell themselves they are not going to have a cake, they find that the urge to eat one becomes overwhelming and they can't wait to have one. Indeed, we can take a great deal of pleasure in the craving for and anticipation of eating our 'forbidden foods'.

If we are made to do without these 'forbidden foods' – particularly if we use them to soothe ourselves – we can become angry, upset and even anxious, and can end up feeling rebellious and resentful. I was watching a TV programme on healthy eating recently and heard that a man of my age should eat a lot less sugar – and yes, you've guessed it: now I really wanted a Jelly Baby, and wanted to tell the well-intentioned presenter to get lost! If we set these rules ourselves we can get into a real pickle, wanting to rebel against the rules, but also beating ourselves up for being so weak as to give in to our cravings – we can't really win sometimes, can we?

There is also a darker side to the emotional associations we can make with food. We can also learn to link certain foods to being rewards that we have to earn, or even punishments that we have to endure (like eating our greens). We can also teach ourselves, or learn from others, that certain foods are bad for us, even disgusting, and become very fearful of eating them, particularly if we are told (as the media often do tell us) that they will make us fat, unhealthy or even just out of step with current fashions.

## The emotions affected by dieting

Many people begin to diet just because they feel they've put on a bit of weight and want to lose it. But many others begin to diet as a way of managing difficult experiences in the past or events that are happening now. These may include losses or major disappointments, bullying, rejection and difficult relationships, which in turn may fuel a desire to be more attractive, or anxiety about health. And, as we saw in Chapter 2, restricting our eating, or even planning to restrict our eating, can have a profound effect on our emotions.

In the early stages of our diet we can experience a significant lift in mood and energy. This can help us feel better if we are feeling low, and even help us feel more confident. Achieving the aim of losing weight, or even just achieving the planned limits on our eating, can also help give us the positive feelings associated with the drive/achievement system. Many people who diet are also concerned about the negative feelings they have about themselves because of their weight or shape, or are fearful of the judgements of others. Setting out to change our weight or shape, particularly if the way we diet is seen by other people, can help us to feel in control of these concerns; it can also help to show other people that we can control our desire for food, and so that we are successful in managing our eating. Diet programmes, TV shows and magazines are full of pictures, stories and tips from 'successful dieters'. Planning to eat less can have a positive effect on our mood, as we anticipate the benefits this will bring us. It can also help to block out more difficult worries or concerns, by giving us something else to focus on that is more in our control.

So there are many reasons why dieting can make us feel good. However, as we also found in Chapter 2, dieting tends to fail after a period of time – in part because of our body's need to eat, but also because dieting tends to create problems of its own, not least of which is the distress caused by having to be constantly vigilant about what we eat.

Of course, many people who overeat do not diet, but even thinking about restricting eating leads to these effects on our mood.

## The social and emotional influences on overeating

As we have seen, eating plays a big part in our social lives. Depending on the situation, sometimes we will eat less in the company of others but at other times we eat more (especially if the occasion involves alcohol as well as food). So social pressure can go either way – to help us moderate our eating or to encourage us to 'have another helping'. We can find it more difficult not to overeat when we are in bigger social groups, particularly if we eat as a way of celebrating or belonging to a group (note that excitement/drive system). Indeed, as I've already noted, overeating is often encouraged and we can find ourselves eating more than we need to in order to go along with others and 'fit in'.

Many of us will know people who encourage us to overeat. They may do this for any or all of a range of reasons, including using food to show their love and affection, because they feel we are undernourished, or because they see making us eat as some sort of competition or battle, even as a way of keeping us dependent on them. Supermarkets and television advertising put a great deal of pressure on us to eat more. Many food manufacturers have increased their portion sizes over the years and increased the amount of sugar and fat in our foods, and 'two for one' and 'eat what you want' promotions are increasingly common. In fact, everywhere you look you can see encouragements to overeat.

People who overeat also tend to be less aware of the messages their bodies give them about when to eat and when to stop. Again, our changing social lives can make it even more difficult to notice these messages. In today's Western culture food tends to be eaten on the go or in front of the TV, and for many of us eating has become a mindless activity. Drinking alcohol while we eat, which is also very common in our society, can also distract us from the signals our body is trying to give us that we have eaten enough.

We have also become a less active society. Many of our jobs do not require much physical activity nowadays; but we are neither eating less, nor doing more physical activity in our leisure time, to take account of this. If anything, we tend to consume more calories as a society than we used to. We now live in a 'super-size' culture, less in touch with our body's signals and having been taught that we should want more than we actually need. All of these social factors can play a role in patterns of overeating.

Attempts to 'solve' this problem have centred on the rise of the diet industry coupled with the belief that being overweight is both a moral and a medical problem. People who are even a little overweight are often demonized. The weight fluctuations and dietary habits of celebrities can be a source of national gossip and often scorn. Jokes about people's weight are socially acceptable, as is the very real discrimination that overweight people can experience. It is not surprising that many of us will diet to lose weight, or just feel so bad about our bodies that we can't see the point in doing anything to improve our health or eating. Sometimes we can even overeat to punish ourselves for being in some way morally inadequate because we cannot meet society's expectations about what our bodies should look like. It is very sad that our children are not immune to these pressures. Their problems with eating can often begin very early in life.

Children as young as eight can feel bad about their bodies and eating, even if they are perfectly healthy, at a normal weight, and eat what they need.

Sometimes overeating can be a form of rebellion again these social pressures. We've already noted that many people diet as a way of managing difficult experiences, either past or present: for a smaller number of people, overeating may be a way of trying to deal with painful events in their past, such as physical, sexual or emotional abuse, bullying or bereavement. A research study I was involved in suggested that at least half the people who come to NHS weight loss clinics are experiencing a degree of psychological distress that would warrant professional treatment. These problems included depression and anxiety, but also worries about size and shape at levels similar to those found in clients with a diagnosis of an eating disorder.

Being distressed, for any reason, can make it more difficult for us to control our eating, even if we are not limiting our food intake. Overeating, or even anticipating overeating, can actually help us to cut off from some of our emotions, and may even give us a sense of pleasure that we may not be experiencing elsewhere in our lives.

## Overeating, rules and self-criticism

Many people who overeat have a lot of rules about eating. These rules tend to develop over time and are personal to them, relating to their own personal histories and hopes and fears around eating. Some of these rules are driven by fear that something bad will happen when you eat; others are based on the hope that eating will help you in some way. Other rules we learn directly from the messages with which the media bombard us every day.

These rules on their own are unlikely to motivate us to comply with them, so we tend to associate them with either a good or a bad outcome (such as 'If I overeat people will think I am greedy' or 'If eat less I will be healthier') and with high levels of emotion (such as fear of failure or anticipated pleasure from achievement). These rules can also conflict with each other, leaving us very confused about how to behave!

Often we are not aware of these rules until we break them. When this happens we can find ourselves overwhelmed with a rush of emotion, often accompanied by anxiety-provoking thoughts, images or memories. Our rules tend to be plausible, even if we often exaggerate the consequences of breaking them. They will make sense for us, because they are based on our personal histories and our hopes for the future, and it can be very hard for any of us to be rational about our rules when we are caught up in the strong feelings they are linked with. It takes a very brave person to ignore their rules to test whether their predictions of what will happen then really come true.

We will explore your own rules about eating, and how you respond if you break an eating rule, in Chapter 7. For now we will explore how these kinds of rules can affect various individuals' eating and emotions by looking at the stories of David, Ann and Alan.

## Eating rules in action

David is typical of many people caught up with rules about eating. He ate a reasonable diet and led a very active life, and his weight was stable. Then, sadly, he became quite ill. Over the course of the next year, while he was unwell, he gradually put on four stone. He became very concerned about this and, as he recovered from his illness, decided that he was going to eat less. David set up many rules about eating, such as 'I must not overeat or I will get fat and have a heart attack, or get cancer again'. His key message to himself was that if he did not keep to a very strict diet his illness would come back. David became very afraid that if he did not lose weight quickly he would become so ill that he would never be able to work again and might even die. Of course, these thoughts were frightening enough to motivate David to limit his eating, and he very rapidly lost weight. As time passed, though, he had strong urges to overeat and after a couple of months he lapsed and broke his diet. Full of self-recriminations, he forced himself back on to his diet until the same thing happened again. David followed this pattern of yo-yo dieting, driven by fear and self-recrimination, for the next ten years.

Sadly, Ann had a difficult upbringing. She lost her father at an early age, and did not find it easy to make friends. She found that eating could be a real comfort to her and gradually came to believe that only food could make her feel better. She had a lot of rules about when she should eat, such as 'I must eat when I want to or I will go crazy', and would often hoard food to make sure that she never ran out. She feared that if she could not eat when she was upset her feelings would become overwhelming and she would end up in a psychiatric hospital.

Alan told me that food was always used as a treat in his family. He was an only child, and remembered with a great deal of affection how his parents and grandparents would always give in to his demands for sweets. There were very few boundaries for him, particularly around eating at meal-times. He couldn't ever recall being told that he was not allowed to eat something the moment he wanted it. He had never learned to use his appetite to regulate his desire for food; instead, he believed that if he did not eat whenever he wanted to it meant he was being deprived or hurt in some way. Alan often got into a battle with himself when he tried not to overeat. He had two sets of rules: one was organized around the belief that he should limit his eating because of his health, the other around the belief that he should eat whatever and whenever he wanted, and if he couldn't do this it meant he wasn't caring for himself. The tension between these two sets of rules often led him to be very distressed when he ate anything, and he became very critical of himself because of his difficulties with eating.

The idea of 'rules' sounds very formal, but all these rules are tied up with important emotions. For example, because Alan had never been limited in his eating, the emotions he associated with limiting his food were those of deprivation, not those of compassionate helpfulness. This sense of deprivation was associated with a range of other painful feelings, including anger, frustration and helplessness, making it very difficult for him to see and experience taking control of his diet as being kind and helpful to himself.

## Rules and self-criticism

You can see that David, Ann, and Alan didn't create the difficulties they experienced around eating; they arose as a consequence of their personal experiences and attempts to manage their lives in the best way they could and were certainly not their fault! Their stories show how our relationship with food can be affected by social and emotional factors and how we can develop a lot of rules to help us manage our relationship with food.

Rules can be a helpful guide for how we should manage our lives and relationships; indeed, without them life would become very chaotic and unpredictable. The problem with rules is that if they are too rigid we are likely to break them. This can cause us a great deal of distress, because when we break our own rules we can often be very self-critical of our inability to keep to them. This is often because we are trying to encourage ourselves to do something that we believe will help us to feel better, so we can tend to see our inability to keep to our eating rules as a sign that we are weak, bad or inadequate.

Marie was typical of many people who overeat. Although she was not actually dieting, she had two competing rules about eating. The first was that she should keep a strict control over eating sweets or other 'junk' food, and that if she could not do this she would become fat and be bullied like her sister was. However, she also believed that chocolate helped her to feel better if she was upset. So she spent her time oscillating between avoiding and craving sweet food. She allowed herself to eat sweet food to fit in with people (for example, if someone brought a birthday cake into work), or if she felt low; but if she did, her initial experience of pleasure though eating was rapidly washed out by the shame and guilt associated with breaking her rule. She tended to call herself names after eating sweet food, and would feel disappointed, angry and even contemptuous of herself. She would then become self-critical and tell herself harshly to 'get back on the straight and narrow'. She often became angry with others for tempting her, and very angry with herself for being so weak in the face of temptation. Occasionally she would get sick of her rules and have a 'stuff it' day, when she ate as much chocolate and sweets as she wanted to help her deal with the misery of daily resisting temptation.

Marie was caught between two parts of herself: one that was condemning and critical, and one that was angry and rebellious. These two parts of her would battle it out – and neither of them was particularly helpful to Marie as a whole. Happily, she found a more helpful way of dealing with this conflict – by learning to pay attention to a third aspect of herself, which was compassionate, understanding and kind. In this way she could escape from the constant see-saw between being forced into change by self-criticism and self-dislike and being pushed into breaking out of her restrictions by feelings of anger and rebelliousness.

**SUMMARY**

As we have seen, the relationship between our emotions and food can be very complex. We can learn to experience positive emotions because of the foods we eat, or the associations we have with eating, or not eating; and our culture and social environment can also prompt us into overeating. We can also learn to attack ourselves for the relationships we have developed with food, particularly for overeating, and this self-criticism can in turn make us overeat even more.

In the next chapter we will explore how compassion for these dilemmas, and for ourselves, can help us to develop a healthier and less distressing relationship with food and eating. We will look at how to manage feelings of distress, how to deal with our desires, and particularly how to manage the self-critical spirals that many people who overeat find themselves in. We will also see how compassion can also help us learn to resist the social pressures we all experience that affect our eating and help us with the struggle with food that many of us face.

# 4 The compassionate mind

In the previous chapter we explored how our relationship with food and eating can be very tricky to manage in today's Western cultures. In the following chapters we will explore our personal relationship with food and eating in more depth, and suggest practical ways to develop eating patterns which will help us to manage overeating. Now, at this point you may have the urge to skip straight to Chapter 12 in an understandable rush to 'do something'. However, please do bear with me for just a while longer. We have already seen that people who have any kind of difficulties with food and eating are often very critical of themselves, and that this self-criticism can make the problems worse. What we are working towards is a compassionate mind approach, which helps us recognize our self-criticism and to disengage from it. When we can do this, we are on our way to taking long-term responsibility for our bodies, rather than just criticizing ourselves into short term-compliance with yet another eating plan!

To do this, obviously, we need to be clear about what we mean by 'compassion' and the 'compassionate mind' approach. So in this chapter we will explore the nature of compassion itself. The ones that follow will guide you through some exercises to introduce you to the skills and practice of self-compassion, before we move on to considering how this compassion approach can be applied to your relationship with food and, specifically, to overeating.

## What is compassion and why is it important?

Many spiritual traditions have suggested that compassion plays a key role in being able to develop happy relationships with other people and happiness within ourselves. According to Buddhist beliefs, over 2,500 years ago in India the Buddha came to realize that our minds are often chaotic, under the push and pull of various desires and wants, and that these are a source of deep unhappiness. This is because we can't always fulfil them, and even if we can it doesn't always lead to good outcomes. As we have already seen, simply eating anything we want when we want (as is now possible in our modern environment) is a recipe for problems.

The Buddha's solution to such difficulties of wanting, craving and attachment to things was the development of two key qualities of mind. The first is *mindfulness* – the development of a clearer, more observant awareness of how our minds work. This includes understanding how our minds create different thoughts, feelings, urges and desires within us. By learning to 'pay attention', in this moment and without judgement, to 'stand back' from and observe the changing climates of our minds (with the arising and passing of feelings and desires, fears and hopes) we can gradually learn to see these patterns of feelings and desires for what they are and as a result to make better choices about what we do: which feelings we will act on and which we will not act on. There are now many books on mindfulness and an increasing number of places where one can learn more about it and practise on retreats or under supervision. We will touch on the basics of mindfulness a little later.

The second key quality of mind identified by the Buddha, and the one that is central to our approach in this book, is *compassion*. Indeed, mindfulness is a way of helping us develop compassion by helping us to recognize that some of our motives, intentions and feelings are not in the best interests of ourselves or others.

At its simplest, Buddhism defines compassion as openness to the suffering of ourselves and others, linked to a commitment and motivation to try to reduce and alleviate that suffering. In order to alleviate suffering, we need to understand its nature. The 'compassionate mind' approach taken in this book acknowledges a debt to Buddhist thinking, and places these aspects centrally in its view of compassion. However, it also turns to new scientific thinking about our minds – how they work and are influenced by different processes which are linked to the way our brain has evolved.

The Buddha outlined a whole programme of living, which he called the eightfold path, geared to being compassion-focused in the way we think, behave, and act towards others. Now, the approach to compassion we're going to take here overlaps quite a lot with the Buddha's notion of the eightfold path, but with a very important additional aspect. This is rooted in the fact that we are all evolved beings – products of the flow of life on this planet. As such we have evolved to need to be cared for from the day we are born to the day that we die. Feeling cared for by others – by our parents, friends, lovers, partners and even our doctors – has a huge impact on how our brains, bodies and minds work. So does feeling cared for by ourselves – self-compassion. There is now very good research evidence showing that developing compassion for ourselves and for others is of great benefit to our mental performance, our emotions, the quality of our relationships, and our abilities to understand and cope with difficult feelings and desires.

## Different states of mind

We've all had the experience of being in different states of mind – being angry or calm, excited or low. We can call an overall state of mind a 'mindset'. For example, we can be in a compassionate mindset or a threatened mindset. The type of mindset that we are in will affect a whole range of ways in which our minds work. It will direct our attention, focus how we think, urge us to behave in certain ways, texture the emotions that flash through us, influence what we're motivated to do and even affect the things we fantasize, dream or ruminate about. To show how this works, Figure 4.1 sets the threatened mind alongside the compassionate mind: as

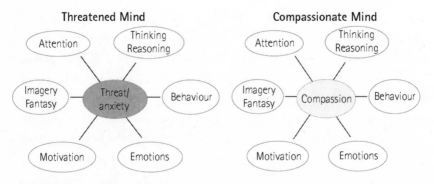

**Figure 4.1:** Two types of mind

*Source*: Adapted with permission from P. Gilbert, *The Compassionate Mind* (London: Constable & Robinson, 2009).

you can see, the six bubbles surrounding the central bubble are the same in both cases; only the core is different. So, for example, the threatened mind will generate one kind of emotions, while the compassionate mind will generate another kind.

Let's explore the concept of different types of mindset, because it is a key idea in terms of learning to develop a compassionate mind. Imagine that you are going for a job interview. This kind of event is naturally likely to get your threat system activated. Remember, your threat system is easy to activate as it's there to detect threats and help you respond quickly to them or avoid them. So even before the interview our threatened mind is working for us – and it may well start to switch on an anxious pattern. Let's look at this pattern by going around the circle in Figure 4.1, starting at the top left-hand bubble.

In an anxious pattern, what are the things we attend to and focus on? We may well be focusing on what the other people will be like. How will the interviewers be with me – will they be friendly or challenging? We might have intrusive images or thoughts about previous occasions, perhaps when things have not gone too well.

How are we thinking and reasoning? Are we reminding ourselves that we've prepared a really good presentation and thinking how impressive it might be? If we're anxious, that's unlikely; it is more likely that we are thinking we might not come over very well, reasoning that as we're anxious we might not present ourselves at our best and that the interviewers might take a rather dim view of us; or that someone else is bound to do better than us and get the job. So our thinking and reasoning are focused on the possible threats in the situation.

What about what our body wants to do? How does it want us to behave? Now, you may want to go to that job interview because you need the job, because it would be a step up, because it means a move to somewhere you want to go – any of the potential payoffs. However, another part of you would rather not have to face it and wants to avoid going. Indeed, if you suffer from a lot of shyness and anxiety you might even have not applied for the job in the first place, despite any or all of these reasons for wanting

hen our threatened/anxious mindset is running the show it can fill
h strong urges to run away or avoid things.

The emotions of our anxious mindset can be simple or complex. If it is only anxiety we feel, then that is reasonably straightforward, but sometimes it's mixed with wanting to engage, so that our positive desires are pulling against the protective ones of avoidance. Indeed, the more badly we want something the more anxious we often are! Sometimes, when we get anxious about things we would like to do, we can be angry with ourselves for getting anxious, for example getting annoyed or disappointed with ourselves for feeling shy in certain situations. We can become angry with our anxiety because we feel that it's holding us back, or that we are somehow different from other people. You can imagine that getting angry with ourselves gives an extra stimulus to our threat system. We now have two threat emotions to cope with: anxiety and (self-directed) anger – certainly not a soothing mixture!

The same potential for conflict applies to our motives – our basic desires, wants and wishes. There can be two types of motive: one relating to our immediate feelings and circumstances (wanting to get away from this threatening situation), and another relating to the longer term (wanting a better future). Our immediate motivation under the pressure of anxiety may be to run away or avoid the threat – after all, our threat system is set up to reduce anxiety by removing us from any possible threat as quickly as possible. It's simply the way our brains are built. Afterwards, we may well feel sad, because we've missed an opportunity – and that can, once again, lead us into self-recrimination and self-criticism.

Last but not least are the images, fantasies and daydreams we create in our minds. These complete the circle, for they are linked to attention. When we become anxious we may have fleeting images of anxious memories or future possibilities. For example, if we are anxious we might create a picture in our minds of sitting on a chair in front of the interview panel feeling anxious and a bit dumbstruck and looking awkward, while the interviewers look at us with stern faces.

So our threatened/anxious mindset pulls on different aspects of our minds to create a pattern – and the different elements of this pattern feed each other. For example, the images that we create in our minds will affect our attention, our thinking, our feelings and how our bodies work. The way we think and reason about what is making us anxious will affect our attention, our feelings, our motivation and our behaviour. This is why we can call the whole thing an 'anxious mindset', because it is about many aspects of the mind working together – with a common single focus on trying to deal with what we perceive to be a threat. The fact that these elements can feed off one another is important: your thinking can drive your anxiety feelings and your anxiety feelings can in turn drive more anxious thoughts, all of which pushes you along the road to more overall anxiety. And all of this happens, remember, because of the way our brains have evolved to live in conditions very different from those of the present. Thanks to evolution, we have brains that are very tricky to live with today!

Fortunately, there is an antidote to the anxious mindset that we can work on developing – the compassionate mind. This mindset is based on understanding and caring and therefore will be more likely to activate the third of our emotional systems, the 'soothing' system, which, as we saw in the previous chapter, is a natural counter to the threat system. The kinder and more understanding we are, the easier it is to tone down the sense of threat that drives this spiral of increasing anxiety.

As well as the more general types of mindset, such as the 'threatened mind' and the 'compassionate mind', we develop more particular types of mindset in responding to particular types of problem. Let's take a look now at some of the most common mindsets that develop around food and eating.

## Food and our states of mind

### The dieting mindset

If you have struggled with your eating for a while it is likely that you have tried to change your 'see-food-and-eat-it' mind into a dieting one. The dieting mind has two elements: it tends to see certain foods both as desired and also as potential threats, and it also tends to focus on the achievements that dieting will bring us. Thus it tends to activate both our threat and our achievement/drive systems.

## Food as threat

For most people who diet, the threat will be one of weight gain. This means that, for many people, food itself becomes a threat because overeating interferes with the real or imagined positive consequences of controlling their weight. Of course, if this is the case your mind will organize itself in ways to help you avoid the threat that eating poses.

In this mindset certain foods in particular tend to be seen as threatening, because they have become associated with weight gain or triggering overeating. They threat they pose may be related to their calorie content or to other nutritional qualities (such as carbohydrate, fat or sugar content). However, the allocation of 'threat' is not always a purely logical decision: sometimes we see a food as a threat because it makes us feel full up or we enjoy its taste, and we associate these feelings with weight gain or the risk of overeating, even if it is less likely to lead to weight gain than other foods we have eaten that day.

If you are in this mindset, and certain foods have become a 'threat', you will learn to pay attention to food in ways that people who don't diet are not really aware of. You may know the fat, calorie, carbohydrate, sugar or fibre content, or glycemic index, of the foods you eat or drink. You may also be very aware of the calories you use when you are active or exercising. You are likely to spend lots of time thinking about eating, and have many rules about what and when you can eat. You are also likely to invest a lot of time and energy in finding ways to avoid overeating. These may include planning and being on a diet, joining diet clubs or programmes to help you manage your eating, and deliberately finding ways to avoid eating (such as not going out for meals with other people). You may become acutely aware of your feelings of hunger in your battle to avoid eating, but you are also more likely to be preoccupied with the smells, tastes and textures of food. You may even dream about eating!

Your 'dieting mind' will also make it easy to remember and think about the problems that overeating may cause you. For example, it may call up painful images of being bullied about your eating or weight, or concerns about your health. You may think that other people will notice and disapprove of your eating and weight; you may imagine that they think you are greedy or out of control of your eating; you may even spend a lot of time comparing how and what you eat to what other people eat – or constantly compare your body size with others, or be particularly attentive to 'how people look' in real life or in magazines and the media.

## Achievement through weight loss

Most people in the dieting mindset will also become very engaged with their drive and achievement system. As we saw in Chapter 2, the drive system gives us good feelings when we pursue things we want or succeed in getting them. This can be true for dieting. The problem here is that the drive system is a double-edged sword. On the up side, when you manage to keep to your diet you get a buzz of pleasure and feel good about yourself – you feel that you are in control and succeeding. Indeed, your biological responses to restricting your eating have actually evolved to give you this boost to your drive system to help you deal with famine, particularly in the early weeks of eating less. So at first you get a 'double whammy': success in doing something you hope will improve your life, and the biological buzz from dieting. This can make you feel great!

To boost these positive feelings, we may provide ourselves with many opportunities to check on and experience this success, such as frequently weighing ourselves, sharing our dieting success with others, planning for the good things that we imagine will happen when we lose weight – for example, buying new clothes – even comparing our own success with the failed diets of others.

Of course, it is understandable that you want these positive feelings, and for a while they can even calm down your 'threatened' dieting mind. However, if you start to struggle to keep to your diet, if you feel low for some reason and resort to comfort eating, if you start going out more often and having a good time and eating more – or if you just get fed up and decide to rebel, then these positive feelings can quickly dry up. When we have tried for something and then fail or suffer a setback, the baulked drive system can switch on the threat system and in come all those familiar sinking feelings – disappointment, frustration, even anxiety.

So then you criticize yourself and try to force yourself back on to your diet. And lo and behold, if you have a few successes you start to feel better again, get that initial buzz again, and the self-criticism and self-dislike die down. But of course, it probably won't be any easier to sustain this time around – so you will experience setbacks, the weight creeps on again, as does the disappointment and frustration – and you're back on the merry-go-round.

You can see how these two aspects of the dieting mindset can work together in Figure 4.2.

So, although on the one hand feeling good about achievements can be helpful, on the other hand we need to be very careful about relying on it.

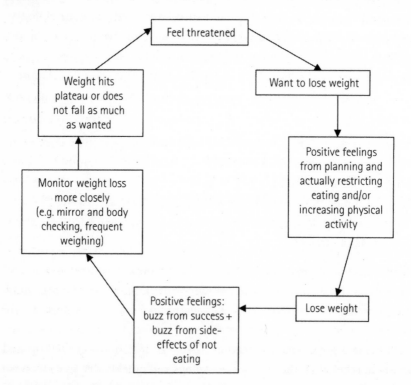

**Figure 4.2:** The dieting mindset

This can be one of the problems with slimming groups, which may overstimulate the drive system by being very positive about success and in so doing increase the chances of overeating or mood problems when people fail. It would be interesting to know, for example, how many people leave these potentially supportive groups because they feel ashamed that they can't maintain their weight-loss targets.

## The comfort food mindset

Another state of mind associated with overeating is what we can call the 'comfort food mindset'. This kind of mindset aims to help us with painful events, memories and feelings. You may remember from Chapters 1 and 3 that we learn that food is comforting from a very early age, as it is often associated with the warmth and security that being fed by an adult can bring. The comfort food mindset also relies on the changes of mood, whether learned or innate, that we associate with certain foods. In trying to ease our distress, this mindset draws us to the types of food and ways of eating that can either soothe present pain or block out memories of painful feelings. We can be preoccupied with eating as much as possible, over the shortest period of time, of the foods that will help manage our mood. This mindset can also involve a lot of planning, food shopping, and arranging time and space (uninterrupted by others) for overeating. It will remind us of the painful experiences or memories that are causing us distress, and often of our previous failed attempts to manage these problems without food. This kind of mindset will help you to override your sensory feelings of fullness, and instead to focus on the emotional benefits of overeating.

As we saw in Chapter 3, our earliest experiences of eating (that is, suckling) are entwined and infused with feelings of emotional closeness, safety and comfort, as well as the physical alleviation of hunger. We can also draw comfort from what is called 'oral gratification' – the sheer taste and feel of those lovely foods in our mouths. What we want in this mindset is the comfort that comes from the process of eating itself, from the textures and tastes and the act of swallowing, rather than the feeling of fullness from having eaten enough. Comfort eating can help us to deal with a sense of threat, too, because if we're focusing entirely on the sensory experiences of eating our minds are totally occupied and we can't focus on other feelings as well.

This kind of mindset is focused on the short-term alleviation of our pain and distress. Of course, in the long term it is likely to lead to a gain in weight, and may not help us find other ways to manage the challenges we face in life. But when we are in pain we tend to be less aware of these unintended consequences – or, if we are aware of them, we are so desperate to ease our distress that 'comfort eating' feels like our best option.

It is very common for the comfort food mindset to be linked to loneliness. When Carol began to monitor her eating behaviour she noted that she tended to overeat in the evenings when her husband worked late and she was home alone watching the television. It took her a while to recognize that actually she was eating because she was lonely and trying to 'while away the time'. A deeper exploration revealed that, although she loved her husband, she felt somewhat dependent on him and had become rudderless in her own life, feeling that she was 'just drifting'. So she thought carefully about this problem and decided that, rather than just focusing on her eating and waiting for her husband to come home, she would go and do some voluntary work on those evenings where he worked late. She found a group of people to join, which improved her social network and lessened her sense of isolation, giving her a sense of purpose and raising her self-esteem. This is an example of where understanding what emotions are behind our 'comfort eating minds' can generate some very interesting solutions that actually have nothing to do with food! As we will see throughout this book, understanding our relationship with food often requires us to understand our relationships with ourselves and how the many facets of our lives interact.

For the moment, though, you can see that the 'dieting mindset' and the 'comfort food mindset' are both frameworks that our brains create to manage problems in our lives. It is really helpful to see that the way our brains do this – setting up patterns in response to challenges, whether these have to do with eating or managing your emotions – is something they have evolved to do, over many thousands of years, in order to help us survive and thrive. It's not your fault that sometimes, in the modern world, they actually make things more difficult for you! One of the difficult problems in managing these types of mind is that they can exist in us at the same time, although we may pay more attention to one or the other at different times. This can lead us into all sorts of tangles as we try to work out whether to diet or comfort eat, whether to diet to deal with the unintended weight gain that results from comfort eating, or whether to comfort eat to deal with the distress of failing in our diets!

## The 'food as fun' mindset

Of course, we don't only see food as either threat or comfort. As we have seen, eating is often associated with sharing, closeness and having a good time.

Being a good host often means providing food for people. There are literally hundreds of books and television programmes dedicated to cooking and presenting aesthetically pleasing and delicious-tasting foods. There is no doubt that food can play an important role in a whole range of enjoyable social activities. So we can get into problems with eating because we are just enjoying having a good time. We go to the restaurant intending not to have that apple pie after just having steak and chips – but everybody's enjoying themselves and we are one glass of wine the better – so what the hell – let's have a good time!

We often feel our lives are so busy, hurried and stressful that we deserve a good time – we don't want constantly to be thinking about limiting ourselves or denying ourselves. We want to go with the flow and to hell with tomorrow. So the 'food as fun' mindset is rather childlike, wanting to do as it pleases and have a good time.

Now, this type of mindset can actually be a source of pleasure and enjoyment: it's the one that starts looking forward to (say) the weekend, to going out, to what you're going to eat and drink – to what you can have that would be pleasurable. This is not about comfort eating; it is more about our drive/excitement system taking over the show. You might also have noticed that this mindset can get quite irritable if it's told to put down limits – it can take quite a firm grip on the controls and be quite resistant to any thought of constraint.

However, the self-critical mind that is so strong a part of many of us who diet and/or overeat can be especially down on this 'food as fun' mindset the day after. We wake up feeling fat and bloated, maybe with a hangover to boot, and think to ourselves: 'Oh, *why* did I do that? Why don't I just have a little more control?' So the self-criticism kicks in – until the next weekend, when maybe the rebellious childlike mindset says, 'To hell with it – let's have fun!' And so the merry-go-round goes on.

## The 'eat to fit in' or 'affiliative eating' mindset

This type of mindset centres on the positive feelings we get from our natural inclination to be part of a group. Sharing eating can help to bring our affiliative soothing system (which we explored in Chapter 3) into play. The combination of these feelings of belonging and safety with the physical pleasures of eating can be a really powerful factor in leading us into overeating.

This mindset can be associated with the 'food as fun' mindset, but this is not always the case. As we saw in Chapter 2, we can often eat to fit in with others. Now, if people around us are eating a little less than we usually do, we will, unconsciously or deliberately, adapt our eating to fit in with them. The reverse can also be true.

In this mindset we want to fit in with others – so that we are seen as part of the social group, just to go along with the flow, or to make us appear desirable in some way. A good example of this mindset in action is the business lunch or dinner. Often I have been out for a meal after a conference or meeting. Usually this is at the end of the day, when I have already eaten most of what my body needs. What I really want to do is have a light snack and go to bed! But out of my desire to be with people I like, or because I feel they will see me as impolite if I just slip away, I can all too easily end up eating a big meal that my body doesn't really want or need. And of course, if I have a drink or two as well, my resistance just drops like a stone.

Sometimes we eat like this to please the people we love – for example, if our partner has cooked a meal for us, even if we already feel full we may eat it to make them feel appreciated.

This desire to use food to cement social bonds goes back millions of years – but of course, our ancestors didn't find it so easy to feast as often as we do! Like the 'food as fun' mindset, this can lead to self-recrimination in the morning and activate the dieting mindset.

## The 'food as punishment' mindset

This type of mindset may be a little less common, but it will be familiar to some people who overeat. They know that the food or the way they are eating is not good for them, but believe that they don't deserve to be treated any better; they may even use the food, or feelings of discomfort from overeating, to hurt themselves for some reason. Often people who experience this mindset have experienced traumatic or abusive histories and may need professional support to change this relationship with themselves.

## An overview of our mindsets

We can see, then, that there are different mindsets – different parts of us, if you like: the 'dieting' part, the 'comfort-seeking' part, the 'let's have fun' part, the 'one of the gang' part – all of which (and you may well be able to think of others) have the potential to fuel problems with our relationship to food. Looking back to Figure 4.1, we can see how our different mindsets affect the way we attend to things, the way we think about things, the way we behave, how we feel, our motivations, and the kinds of images and fantasies we create. This why, in the compassionate mind approach, we talk about these parts of us as 'mindsets', because they integrate different aspects of our minds. So we use the concept of a 'compassionate mindset' – or, for brevity, 'compassionate mind' – because it helps us to recognize that we're dealing with an integrated style of thoughts, feelings, how we pay attention to things, what we want to do and so on.

The other central point to remember all the time is that these mindsets or parts of ourselves, which cause us difficulties with our eating behaviour, arise mostly because of the kinds of lives we lead in the modern Western world – and I want to keep stressing this: for it is only in the modern Western world that it has become so easy to obtain foods that have been artificially enhanced in colour, taste and texture specifically to stimulate our appetites and to act as a source of comfort.

As we begin to understand in detail the key issues that lie behind our eating difficulties, we will come to see more and more clearly why we need to develop our compassionate mind so that, working with these other mindsets, we can take responsibility, with wisdom and understanding, for our own bodies – and learn to live contentedly and healthily with our 'see-food-and-eat-it' brain in our modern world.

## Shifting towards a compassionate mind

It can be very helpful to learn to become more aware of how our threatened mind works, and, if we are overeating, to understand in particular our dieting and comfort food mindsets. As we become 'mindful' of these patterns and come to recognize how they are driven by the threat or achievement/excitement systems, we can also learn to take steps to activate a different type of mind – one driven by the contentment/soothing system. This in turn can help us to learn to manage our 'see-food-and-eat-it brain', and to deal with the painful challenges of life and the pressure to 'just to enjoy ourselves regardless' or eat to fit in.

As we will see, the compassionate mind is never critical but always understanding of the difficulties of modern living and of the complexities and hardships we face. However, it is by no means passive. It is focused on and develops our inner wisdom. It is motivated to work in our best interests, to do things that are genuinely caring and to help us to develop a sense of well-being in the long term. Compassion takes the long view about our health and happiness, looking over and beyond just having a good time on a particular day or just eating to get rid of feelings on that day. Compassion always seeks the 'middle way' and avoids rigidity and black-and-white decisions or behaviours – such as those inflexible dieting rules.

There is another reason why cultivating compassion is helpful, and this is related to how our three emotional systems interact. Although, as we saw in Chapter 3, different types of feeling can sometimes coexist (we can be anxious and excited at the same time, or angry with people we love), harnessing one type of feeling tends to reduce feelings of other types – at least for a time. In the West a group of psychotherapists called behaviour therapists (who focus on changing our behaviour) came to realize that we can learn to generate one emotion to dissipate another. They first focused on anxiety and suggested that the state of relaxation could not coexist with the state of high anxiety. This led to the development of relaxation training. So now many therapists teach anxious people ways to relax – and indeed, help people to develop different feelings by creating certain states of mind – through imagery, relaxation, body work or even dance. The point here is that learning to develop the compassionate mindset can reduce the power of our threatened, dieting and comfort food mindsets and help us to find other ways to deal with the challenges of life. Equipped with a compassionate mind, we are better able to take responsible and wise decisions that genuinely are in our best interests and support our well-being in the long term.

## Our compassionate mind: an overview

Now, before you read this section you might like to stop and look again at the outline of the compassionate mind in Figure 4.1 (page 70). We are now going to take a quick tour round the circle to see what each of the six aspects means in the context of the compassionate mind.

*Compassionate attention* will turn to helpful, supportive memories and a positive focus. Let's imagine that sometimes you overeat to comfort yourself for a lack of confidence; perhaps you feel uncertain about how other people see you or whether they like you. Your threatened mind will focus on the times when things didn't seem to go well – that's its job, of course, to bring the threat to your attention – further encouraging your 'comfort eating' mindset. Your compassionate mind, on the other hand, will direct attention to times when you have been successful, times when you have got on well with other people, and will prompt you to remember the times when people have been kind.

*Compassionate thinking and reasoning* focus on understanding that overeating is a very common problem, and we all suffer from it to greater or lesser degrees because evolution has given us very tricky brains and bodies to deal with – *not* because of some moral failure on our part: this is an important compassionate insight. It is also important to recognize how we can overeat either accidentally or deliberately, and how our biological impulses and responses around eating developed because they gave us an evolutionary advantage.

*Compassionate behaviour* is working out and taking actions which are in our best interests and, of course, the best interests of others. Sometimes this is fairly straightforward, but sometimes it may require us to develop courage and learn how to engage with things even when we are frightened of doing so or they are difficult. Compassionate behaviour might also involve learning more about our eating and practising different ways of coping with our feelings and nurturing ourselves. Thus we can learn ways to manage our emotions and our see-food-and-eat-it brain that will help us develop a healthier and happier relationship with food. It is very likely that we will need to develop compassionate behaviour 'one step at a time'. It is usually best to practise slowly, and to get skills in place before we need them. This means practising certain things when it's easy to do so. For example, if you're learning to swim, it's not helpful to learn in the open sea in a storm – far better to start off in the shallow end of a warm swimming pool! Sometimes it's hard to face up to things, and if we don't want to think about them we don't practise and prepare ourselves. Compassionate behaviour is about kindly encouraging ourselves to do those things that are in our long-term best interests, even if it is uncomfortable in the short term.

*Compassionate emotions* are linked to feelings of warmth, support, kindness and belonging. If you try to give yourself encouraging thoughts, are you able to hear those in your mind with kindness and warmth? For example, if you're going to an interview and you think to yourself, 'I have done this before, and if I don't get the job I'll be disappointed but I can cope,' do you hear that in a genuinely kind and concerned tone, or in a kind of 'pull yourself together and stop being silly and getting into a state' tone? The emotions that we generate by talking to ourselves can affect how helpful our thoughts are. So it is helpful to create compassionate tones and feelings in our minds when we are being supportive. The next chapter will introduce some exercises that, with the help of compassionate images, will enable you to practise this, and there are further exercises along these lines throughout the book.

*Compassionate motives* are at the core of our idea of compassion. These are the desire and intention to relieve suffering, both in yourself and in others, and to behave in ways that genuinely enable you to flourish in the long term and support your own and others' well-being. Now, you might think that the best way to relieve suffering if you're anxious is simply to avoid the things that make you anxious – no more anxiety then! The problem is that this sets up another source of suffering, for if you have been anxious about going for something you wanted, then you have not been able to achieve your goal. Also, avoidance cuts down your options and increases the chances that you will feel anxious again. So, rather than learning how to deal with the anxiety, you get stuck with it. To make progress here we have to be honest with ourselves: to really think about our values and the kind of person we want to be (or become), and how to bring that about. In relation to overeating, compassionate motivation involves harnessing the inner desire to reduce our suffering and act in ways that generally support our well-being, whether this be tackling overeating itself or its consequences, such as weight gain.

*Compassionate images* are supportive, understanding, kind and encouraging. When we are anxious it is very easy to generate frightening images or even self-critical ones. But we can train ourselves to deliberately create different types of images in our minds and in this way stimulate different brain systems – especially the soothing/contentment system. Again, the exercises introduced in the next chapter will help you learn to create this supportive kind of image and to practise calling these images up when you need them.

## Our compassionate mind: the bigger picture

We are now ready to explore in a little more detail what we mean by a 'compassionate mind'. Why would we want to be compassionate, and where do our desires and abilities to be compassionate come from? These are interesting questions. The short answer is that they come from our motives and capacities to be caring. For example, as a species of mammal we give birth to live babies whom we look after and nurture. Evolution has given us protective and caring feelings towards our children. We enjoy seeing them grow and we become unhappy if they are unhappy or distressed or hurt. Additionally, we have caring feelings for the other people around us such as siblings, parents, friends and colleagues. Their emotional states affect ours. We may even be affected by the distress or happiness of someone little known to us.

The reason why evolution gave us these motivations and feelings is complex, but basically it boils down to the fact that humans and other animals that are motivated to help each other survive and reproduce better than those who are not. This doesn't mean that at times we are not very selfish, critical and cruel – clearly we have those potential mindsets in us too. It is important to recognize that our brains have programmed into them a host of different potential states of feeling and thought. It is our responsibility to understand these and equip ourselves to choose which ones we want to activate.

Interestingly, it is usually when the threat system raises its head that we are likely to turn away from caring. We are less likely to have caring feelings for people we're frightened of, or who we feel are more powerful than us, or whom we don't like. Our attitudes towards these people are often wary and defensive, and that of course turns off our interest in compassionate caring. We fight our enemies rather than caring for or about them.

As we will see later, the same is true when it comes to relating to and thinking about ourselves. If we are angry with and critical of ourselves, that tends to turn off our caring and soothing motivation and feelings towards ourselves – the very systems that could help to combat the threat system.

As I said, the reasons why these motives and feelings arose are complex; fortunately, we don't need to worry too much about their origins, apart from understanding that they evolved over many thousands of years. What we do need to do is understand them and then learn to harness them. So now I'm going to introduce you to the 'compassion circle' developed by

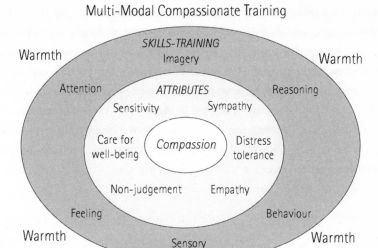

**Figure 4.3:** The compassion circle

*Source*: Adapted with permission from P. Gilbert, *The Compassionate Mind* (London: Constable & Robinson, 2009).

Paul Gilbert, who derived it from the research and ideas of many other people – including, of course, those from various spiritual traditions.

The full circle is given in Figure 4.3. OK, it may look a bit daunting, but in fact we've already gone through a lot of it. You see that the figure separates compassionate attributes (in the middle ellipse) from compassionate skills (in the outer ellipse). The attributes are the qualities that power compassion along, while the skills are the capacities which harness those attributes and through which they are translated into action. We have covered the skills in the previous section, so here we will focus on the attributes.

## Compassionate attributes

### Care for well-being

Let's begin on the right-hand side of the middle ellipse, where you can see 'care for well-being'. This attribute captures the motivation to be caring; the decision and commitment that you do wish to relieve suffering (in yourself and others). This might be a place to begin to look at the advantages and disadvantages of becoming compassionate: to think about what you have to lose in trying; to see if perhaps you feel you couldn't do it so you've decided against it already – 'What's the point?' you say. Or maybe you feel that you have so many angry or other unpleasant thoughts and fantasies that you can't imagine being caring. Well, all humans have difficult feelings and fantasies, and this does not make you in any way less able to be caring, though it might mean you will need to focus on developing this attribute.

## Sensitivity

Moving one place clockwise round the middle ellipse, we come to 'sensitivity'. This means being open to what's going on in and around you; learning to pay attention and notice when you or others are in distress or are experiencing certain emotions. Sometimes when we feel distressed we try not to notice it – we try to avoid our feelings because we 'don't want to go there'. Sometimes when we overeat we don't want to think about the feelings that might be associated with what we're doing; or we might become angry with ourselves ('Oh gosh, here I go again! *Why* do I eat so much? What's the matter with me? Why can't I be like other people?!') rather than being sensitive, gentle and understanding. Many of us say unpleasant things to ourselves that we wouldn't dream of saying to another person who struggles with their eating. If we're honest, we lack sensitivity to our see-food-and-eat-it brain.

## Sympathy

Next around the circle is sympathy. Some people think that sympathy is a bad thing: it's like indulging oneself or feeling sorry for oneself or, even worse, 'pitying' oneself – or others. That is a big misunderstanding of sympathy. Sympathy is simply the ability to be emotionally moved. Suppose you see a three-year-old child happily walking down the street. You may smile at her happiness – but then she trips over the kerb and bangs her head heavily and is hurt. Her laughter turns to tears as she experiences real pain. You are likely to feel a flash of sadness and anxiety, and to want to rush out and make it better. Sympathy is that emotional connection to pain – it arises without thinking, moving us immediately. Developing sympathy for ourselves can sound more difficult, but it's the same principle. So, with wisdom, we can learn to be sensitive and open to our difficulties and also moved by our them.

## Distress tolerance

If we are aiming to cultivate sympathy and the ability to be moved by suffering, it may seem strange that we should 'tolerate' distress. In fact, this is a very important attribute. Here's why. When the 'threat system' is in control, it pushes us into avoidance – away from unpleasant feelings that are threatening us. This is what it is designed to do; but the trouble is, if we always shy away from painful or frightening emotions, and situations that ignite them, we never learn that those difficult feelings are in fact bearable and that we can learn how to cope with them and the situations that provoke them. And the more we avoid the unpleasant feelings or situations, the more we feel that we could never cope with them and so the more anxious we become about them. On the other hand, if we learn to accept the difficult feelings – kindly, gently, uncritically – we learn both that they are not in fact unbearable and that there are ways to cope with them. So learning how to tolerate our urges to overeat and our desires for food without acting them out (even postponing them for just a short time), and noticing how we can stay with our feelings without taking action, can be very important in helping us cope with them. We are learning to tolerate, as opposed to act on, our feelings. Learning to be mindful and observant – having sensitivity – can help us with tolerating distress. Learning to be more empathic and less judgemental (the next two attributes) will also help us.

You can see how this works in practice if you think of a child who is anxious about going out with other children. Researchers have found that many anxious children have anxious parents. So if the child becomes anxious about going to a party with other children they don't know very well, the parent might let them stay at home so they won't be anxious any more. Unintentionally they're teaching their child a number of things. One is that painful emotions are not to be faced and dealt with, but are best avoided; another is that painful emotions can be overwhelming. Because the child did not go to the party they won't become familiar with the children they didn't know, and so next time there's a party with those children, what are they likely to do? Yes – feel even more anxious and want to avoid it again. Sadly, while only wanting to protect their children, these parents are not helping the children to understand how their minds work, or how to face up to and cope with difficult feelings and situations – which is a skill they will need in their future lives. It is tough to tolerate distress, but as you can see, compassion is not about avoidance – it's about doing those things that are genuinely helpful in the long term, and doing them kindly, gently and without harsh criticism.

Another reason distress tolerance is very important is because sometimes people think that compassion is about soothing painful feelings away – getting rid of them. Now, of course, sometimes we can soothe painful feelings away, but that's not always possible or even desirable. If we are very angry about something we may need to learn how to deal with the anger: to be honest about our feelings and learn to be assertive. Compassion is not about avoiding addressing issues. Sometimes we have to learn how to tolerate powerful feelings and fantasies we don't like – even thoughts of hate. One of the biggest confusions and misunderstandings of compassion is the idea that it's just about 'being nice' and hiding one's feelings or suppressing them. That is not helpful or compassionate, and while brutal honesty all the time is not helpful, neither are suppression and avoidance. Of course, this is not an excuse to be rude or unpleasant, either. There are respectful ways to be assertive and powerful.

## Empathy

Empathy is the uniquely human ability to think about and understand the nature of our minds and those of others. Unlike other animals, we recognize that people do things for reasons: because they are motivated, because they want things and have desires, because they're anxious or angry, because they might not know the full picture – or because of impulses of which they're not even aware. We recognize that people can be mistaken in their views, and have false beliefs. Just as we can understand the minds of others, so we can come to understand our own minds. We can reflect on and think about how our minds work. When we have empathy for our struggles with food and eating we're able to understand the nature of these problems, how they are rooted in the way our bodies and brains have evolved, how our own personal difficulties with overeating may have developed, what situations can make the problem worse, and the kinds of things we do when we feel the urge to overeat, eat unhealthy foods or restrict our eating too much. Empathy is a very important attribute in compassion because it is based on a deep understanding and acceptance of how our minds and bodies work.

## Non-judgement

Last but not least is the attribute of non-judgement. Now, not judging does not mean having no preferences or desires. Indeed, we know that some of our desires and preferences for food are inbuilt. Non-judgement really means non-condemnation; it means letting go of that angry desire to attack and be critical. It is also an essential part of that other key quality of mind that goes along with compassion, as we saw at the beginning of this chapter – mindfulness. The more we ease back from charging in and criticizing, which can sometimes be our immediate reaction to a problem or perceived failing, the greater the chances we have for reflection and thinking about how best to deal with it.

## How it all fits together

You can probably see from this brief tour of the compassionate attributes that they all build on and support one another. So, the more compassionate motivation you build up, the easier it may be to develop the other attributes. Equally the more sensitive and the more empathic you become to your eating difficulties, whatever they may be, the more strongly motivated you will be to deal compassionately with them. In the chapters to come we will be working with this family of attributes to build up the overall compassionate mind approach.

We will also be working on the skills located in the outer ellipse of Figure 4.3. Like all skills, these are learned by practice: so we can train ourselves in (for example) creating and building images that are helpful and compassionate, aimed at stimulating the soothing emotional system; we can train our reasoning and thinking to focus compassionately; we can train ourselves to behave in compassionate ways that are in our long-term interests. We can train our bodies to create compassionate sensations (for example, by using imagery), and we can use our images and other ideas to generate compassionate feelings. Last but not least, we can practise compassionate attention, looking for what is helpful and supportive in and around us, rather than letting the threat system always direct us towards the things we are frightened of or angry about.

### SUMMARY

By now you will have seen how our three inbuilt systems of emotions become involved with eating, and how complex these links and effects can be. Certain foods can be threats; losing weight can become an achievement which gives us good feelings when we feel in control – but then we can get into trouble if we lose control. Eating can be a source of comfort, or a way of rebelling against constraints and rules; a way of belonging to a group and even a way of punishing ourselves.

In the chapters ahead we will see how developing a compassionate mind approach can help us to deal with all these mindsets that can get us into problematic relationships with food. By way of preparing the ground, this chapter has provided an overview of how we see compassion within this compassion-focused approach, and of the various elements that go to make up the compassionate mind. In the following chapters we shall be exploring all of these elements and how they can be applied to helping you to manage overeating.

# 5 Preparing your mind for compassion

The previous chapter outlined the various aspects of the compassionate mind – a mind that is open to our suffering and the suffering of others, and is committed to trying to reduce that suffering. A focus on compassion influences our attention, the way we think and reason, the way we behave, and our emotions and feelings. In the coming chapters we will explore compassionate ways of helping us change our relationship with food, eating and our body towards a healthier balance.

This chapter begins by introducing work with imagery and then sets out some initial exercises that will help you to prepare your mind for a compassionate focus. It then moves on to further exercises that explore ways to develop different specific facets of our compassionate mind. Some of these exercises are like physiotherapy for our brains, stimulating our brains in various ways. Just as our bodies respond to physical exercise by getting fitter and better toned, so research shows that practising self-compassion can affect our brains, increasing positive moods and feelings of self-confidence and thereby benefiting our social relationships. In later chapters we will see how we can use these exercises and basic ideas to help us re-examine our beliefs and change our relationship with food and eating.

As someone who has played a lot of sport and had a lot of sporting injuries, I know that physiotherapy and exercises to get fit or develop sporting skills take time and practice to show their effects. I also know that progress is often best achieved by taking small steps rather than trying to do too much at once, and that sometimes we need to strengthen certain parts of ourselves before we tackle some of the more demanding exercises. It's just the same with the exercises in this book aimed at developing your compassionate mind: the more you practise, the better you'll get, but it's a good idea to take it slowly and not to ask too much of yourself all at once.

Also, as with any new skill, we don't want to be trying to practise under pressure. Ideally, try to practise the skills described in this chapter when you are feeling relatively OK – or at least, not when you are really cross, or miserable, or frustrated with your eating habits. As you get better at using each skill you will gradually be able to incorporate it into your alternative ways of managing discomfort or distress.

## Working with imagery

Images can be very powerful and rapidly activate various systems in our brain. Certain images can stimulate the parts of our brain that help us to feel soothed and safe, and at the same time tone down other emotional systems (especially the threat system) that may be associated with eating difficulties. In this way they can help us to break the association between food and emotional comfort.

Now, people sometimes think that when we try to create images in our minds they should be like photos – clear and sharp. In fact they don't have to be anything like that. Sometimes imagery only gives us a 'sense' of something and we never see anything clearly. So imagery doesn't have to mean fully formed pictures – very often it consists of just fleeting impressions.

People often say they're not particularly visual or good with fantasy. But supposing I say to you the word 'bicycle'. What popped into your head? Now suppose I ask you, 'Where are the brakes on a bicycle?' What pops into your mind now? How does your mind provide you with this information so that you can answer the question? Basically, you're running images in your head – without even trying to.

Now, in working with imagery to develop the compassionate mind we're interested in the way certain images are related to certain feelings and mental states. So, for example, if you have an interview coming up tomorrow and are a bit anxious about it, you might have images and thoughts popping into your head that make you anxious. However, you might take your children to the park, and find that playing with them distracts you from your anxious thoughts and images so that after a while you feel less anxious. Eventually you forget all about tomorrow. But then, after the children have had their tea and are in bed, you're lying in the bath and all of a sudden you remember that tomorrow you've got that interview. In a flash the anxious images pop into your mind again (a stern figure behind a desk, a dark room, the feeling of nervous perspiration on your hands) and up comes the anxiety again. Now, if we imagine the interviewers are going to be very supportive, kind and interested in us, that the room is going to be comfortable and pleasant, we might have a different emotional experience. We are likely to feel far less anxiety than if we imagine they're going to be very tough, aggressive and critical. So the nature of the image will have a major impact on how anxious you feel.

Images that set off our anxiety typically come to us at the end of a hard day, in our dreams, or while we are between sleep and waking. They can even wake us up! But, rather than letting those images, which will influence our feelings, come and go as they please, according to what's going on inside and around us, we can actually turn this ability to fantasize and imagine to our advantage by deliberately choosing images that will stimulate the soothing system rather than (say) the threat system. One way to do this might be to begin by focusing on the feelings of contentment and safeness in a particular place. We call this 'safe place' imagery and will explore how to help you do this a little later in this chapter.

## Choosing what we pay attention to

You may have already noticed that our minds can be quite unruly things. I am doing my best to concentrate on writing the next sections of this book, but I have at least three other things buzzing around in my head, including planning for the weekend, wondering what to cook for dinner, and the tax return that I need to complete tonight! The good news is that this is perfectly normal; our brains have the ability to multi-task. However, we can find it especially difficult to concentrate on one thing if our threat system is very active. In evolutionary terms this makes sense, as we need to pay attention to any threats, so the threat system has evolved to be very good at distracting us from anything else! These days, though, our feelings of threat are quite likely to relate to things that are not a danger to our survival, and we need to learn alternative ways to manage them – including being able to focus our attention where we want it. This can be especially useful in dealing with impulses to restrict our eating, or overeat for comfort, or criticize ourselves for how we are eating.

We're now going to explore two ways of working with your attention. The first is to develop your capacity to be *mindful* of the thoughts and feelings that you experience. The second is to develop your ability to deliberately refocus your attention.

## Mindful attention

There is a very long tradition in Eastern religions, particularly Buddhism, of training attention. The practice of doing this is known as 'mindfulness'. In recent years, Western therapists have discovered that learning to be mindful is extremely beneficial for a range of psychological difficulties and in dealing with the stresses that all of us face to some degree in our lives. Mindfulness is a way of paying attention to the things going on around us and in our own minds. The aim of mindfulness is to be fully in the present in each moment, rather than constantly being pulled away from the present moment with worries, plans and ruminations. Learning to recognize this shifting away from the present moment is key to mindfulness. So the key skill we need to practise in developing it is *the act of noticing the shift and then returning the attention to our desired focus*. Mindfulness is *not* 'making' your mind pay attention or emptying your mind of thoughts. It is noticing the shifting of your mind and then returning it to its focus. As we will see later, this can be very helpful when doing compassion exercises.

A second aspect of mindfulness is noticing how our thoughts and emotions emerge – for example, learning to pay attention to the bodily experiences of wanting to eat and to label them. So we might say to ourselves: 'I'm having the feeling in my body of wanting to eat; I am having fantasies of biscuits and chocolate cakes; I'm feeling the urge to put those in my mouth.' In this way the feelings are no longer just semi-conscious impulses guiding your behaviour; by bringing them into the forefront of your consciousness and paying them attention, you learn to observe them and really know what they feel like. Learning to 'speak the feelings out' like this – putting words to our thoughts, feelings and fantasies – helps us to slow down and to become more observant and more aware of things emerging in our minds and bodies rather than just following our impulses without stopping to consider them.

You might also become aware that when you try to resist the urge to eat, another set of feelings, urges and thoughts will appear in your mind which try to nudge you towards overriding any resistance to eat. These would include the 'stuff it' thoughts, such as 'Oh, stuff it, I want to eat and I'm going to!' or 'Stuff it, I don't want think about this and I'm just going to eat!' You might then follow that thought curiously and wonder where it's come from, what it's about, and what happens if you challenge it. Or, if you have feelings of anxiety about eating, when you become mindful you will pay attention to the anxiety *as an observer* and again be curious about the thoughts that pop into your mind as a result of the anxiety.

So, to be mindful is to become more observant of the ever-changing flow of emotions and thoughts that ripple through our bodies and pop in and out of our minds. Once we have learned to observe these thoughts and feelings, we can begin to make choices about whether to act on them or not. So the key to mindfulness is this slowing-down, paying more attention to the present moment and becoming more observant of the contents of our mind and the feelings in our body. We will explore this approach in the first exercise below; but first we'll take a brief look at another way of training our attention.

## Refocusing our attention

This is somewhat different from mindfulness. It involves learning to use imagery or physical activity deliberately to shift our attention away from the present to a mindset we would prefer to be in. Like summoning up fleeting images, this is something that we do naturally and voluntarily: for example, all of us have probably chosen to daydream about our holidays to take our mind off some rather humdrum or unpleasant task, or to do something that we know will distract us from thinking about something difficult. Later in this chapter we will look at how you can learn to refocus attention to get yourself into a specific mindset, when we explore the idea of a 'safe place' and compassionate imagery. In the next chapter we will also look at more practical ways to use this skill to help us manage the emotions that may arise when we change our eating.

## EXERCISE 5.1: MINDFUL ATTENTION

Sit quietly for a moment and focus on your breathing. Allow the breath to come right down into your lungs slowly and evenly, and then leave your body slowly and evenly. If you find this difficult, you may simply want to try to focus on the sensation of your breath coming in and leaving through your nose. Try spending two minutes simply holding your attention on the experience. If you don't like focusing on your breathing, you could use a pebble or a shell and try to focus your attention on the experience of looking at it and feeling it.

You may notice that within just a few moments your mind will have wandered off on to something else. This happens to all of us: we all have things in our minds, and our attention easily gets pulled towards them and away from the present moment. It happens whether the things in our minds are things that are worrying us (an interview coming up), or things we are looking forward to (like a party), or things that we need to do (pay a bill, or remember to call a friend) – whatever is in our mind, our attention will skip from one to another. This is absolutely typical of how our minds work; indeed, recent research evidence suggests that it is our natural state.

One aspect of practising mindfulness is just learning to notice when your mind wanders and bringing your attention *gently* and *warmly* back to what you want to focus on: that is, not beating yourself up for having a grasshopper brain but kindly and uncritically pointing your attention back to the moment. To repeat: mindfulness is not *making* our mind pay attention or *emptying* our mind of thoughts; and telling ourselves off for not being able to pay attention is not being mindful either! Indeed, it is counterproductive, as it's actually very useful to notice where your mind wanders off to: this will often help you to identify issues that are bothering you. When your mind wanders it is not a sign that you have failed to be mindful, it is just a normal part of the process. It is the act of noticing the wandering and then returning the attention to the desired focus that is central to mindfulness. The very fact that you find this difficult is itself evidence that you are engaging in mindful practice!

You might try to practise this 'mindful attention' exercise for a couple of minutes, three times a day. In the early stages you may only be able to focus your attention for 10–20 seconds at a time. That's fine; remember, the key to mindfulness is to notice where your mind wanders to and gently bring it back to the present moment, focusing on your breathing, or your shell or pebble.

Developing our mindful attention skills can provide us with a useful way to slow down the rush to follow our impulses to eat and help us to notice what drives these impulses. However, I have found that it can be helpful to have a structure for eating in place before we apply mindfulness to the experience of eating, and so we will postpone exploration of eating mindfully until Chapter 13.

## Activating your soothing system

One of the keys to developing self-compassion is learning to turn off, or at least tone down, the 'threat' and 'drive' systems of emotion regulation. If either of these systems is in full flow, it can be very difficult for our compassionate mind to get through. So, the first thing we need to do is to learn how to bring to the fore the third of those emotion regulation systems – the 'soothing' system.

### Soothing breathing rhythm

As we saw in Chapter 3, our threat and drive systems are associated with particular types of physical and emotional responses. The soothing system is also associated with a set of physical and emotional responses: feeling calm, contented, connected and safe. Soothing rhythm breathing is an exercise specifically developed to activate this system. Unlike some relaxation training exercises, it is designed to help you find your own soothing rhythm for breathing, rather than asking you to follow a specific rate or pace. It also includes an element of mindfulness that can begin to develop the skills outlined in the previous section.

### Exercise 5.2: Soothing Breathing Rhythm

Begin by finding a quiet place where you know you can sit without being disturbed for at least ten minutes. Sit in a chair with an upright posture (don't let your head fall forward) and place both feet on the floor about shoulders' width apart. Rest your hands on your thighs.

Begin by gently focusing on your breathing. Initially, just notice the breath going in and out though your nose. As you breathe, notice the air coming down into the bottom of your ribcage. Feel your diaphragm – the area underneath your ribs – move as you breathe in and out. Just notice your breathing and experiment with the pace: breathe a little faster or a little more slowly, and notice the difference in how your body feels. Generally, soothing rhythm breathing is slightly slower and slightly deeper than your normal breathing rhythm. You might start by trying a count of about three seconds breathing in, then a slight pause, then three seconds breathing out – but this is just a guideline to get you going: the point is to find a breathing pattern that, *for you*, seems to be *your own* soothing, comforting rhythm. It is as if you are checking in, linking up, with the particular rhythm within your body that is soothing and calming to you. Whatever comfortable, soothing pace you settle on, try to ensure that your breaths in and out are smooth and even. For example, notice if you're breathing a bit too quickly, snatching a bit tensely at the in-breath or rushing the out-breath.

Now spend 30 seconds or so just focusing on your breathing. Just notice the breath coming down into your lungs towards the diaphragm, the diaphragm expanding, and then the air moving out through your nose. Sometimes it's useful to focus your attention on the point just inside the nose where the air enters.

Even in those 30 seconds you may have noticed that your wandering mind crept in with other thoughts, or that you became distracted by other noises in or outside the room. When you first do this exercise, you might be quite surprised at just how much your mind does shift from one thing to another. This is all very normal, natural and to be expected. When it happens, just notice that the mind has wandered and gently and kindly bring it back to its focus. At all times remember that you're not trying to force yourself to do anything, to clear your mind of thoughts or to make yourself concentrate. You are simply noticing and gently refocusing; noticing and gently refocusing. In this case you are gently (re)focusing on the feelings of your breathing and your body slowing down. You might notice, for example, that you feel your body becoming heavier in the chair.

Remember, we are not aiming to 'achieve' any specific emotional or physical state in this exercise. It is designed simply to help you link into your soothing system and see what happens. Some people report that when they find their own soothing breathing rhythm it helps them to feel calmer, slows their thoughts down and relaxes them. Some people even use this exercise to help them get ready for sleep. These effects can be very helpful – but the central purpose of the exercise is to begin to learn to train our attention by establishing a breathing rhythm that can activate our soothing system. You can use the motto 'notice and return' to guide you: *notice* the distractions and *return* your attention to your breathing. If you have 100 thoughts, or even 1,000 thoughts, that doesn't matter at all. All that matters is that you notice and then, to the best of your ability, gently and kindly bring your attention back to the breathing.

As you practise 'notice and return', you may find that gradually your mind will bounce around less and you will have fewer distracting thoughts. It may become easier to focus your attention on your breathing – but some days it will be easier than others. If you worry that you are not doing it right or that it cannot work for you, then just note these thoughts as typical intrusions and return your attention to your breathing. Remember, the wandering mind is normal, and indeed can provide us with very useful information to work with later on. So don't get angry with it, or become self-critical; just kindly bring your attention back to the focus of your breathing. It is the act of noticing how our minds wander that is the beginning of mindfulness.

You can do these two exercises at any time and in any place; you can even do them standing up (say, on a bus or tube train, or in a queue at the post office). All they require is that you allow yourself a few moments when you focus on your breathing and gently bring your mind back to that single focus when it wanders. The key thing is our mindful attention to the process rather than the result.

One of the key elements of mindfulness is to *remember* to become mindful. We can, of course, spend time deliberately practising mindfulness by focusing on our breathing or some other activity, and indeed at the beginning this is just what we need to do; but actually every moment of our lives could be lived more mindfully. This is an approach that you can use in many aspects of life, and indeed you can practise becoming more mindful in all that you do.

## Developing your 'safe place'

Some of us, when we are distressed, naturally conjure up images of being in a better place, maybe somewhere we remember from the past or somewhere we hope to be in the future. Now, of course, we may do this simply to escape or avoid difficult feelings or situations. However, we can also use this tactic to help us cope with difficult situations *without* avoiding them, because it can help us to learn ways of containing and creating soothing feelings within ourselves.

The 'safe place' exercise builds upon this natural way that people activate their soothing system. The feelings of safeness and calmness it encourages are useful in activating our soothing system; and when this system is engaged it becomes easier to think about our difficulties from a more compassionate perspective and also to experiment with new ways of coping. Developing a safe place does not mean that we either accept or ignore bad things happening to us, or that we do not try to change things in our life. It is simply a step towards feeling calm enough to tackle these things without resorting to overeating as a way of coping with difficult feelings that may arise.

I have found that many people find it easier to develop their safe place when they have a little practice in using soothing rhythm breathing. So we will begin the exercise below with this. If you find that you can get straight into your safe place without this, that is absolutely fine. In compassion focused therapy we are always experimenting, trying out things to find what is *personally* helpful for us.

Some people have clear ideas about places they like or places they feel safe in, but others don't. If nowhere springs to mind for you, it's a good idea to try thinking about the sorts of places you could feel safe in before you do the exercise. So, when you have some space and time to fantasize, ask yourself what sort of a place would make you feel safe. Would it be outside or inside? If outside, what would the weather be like? What colours would there be around you? Remember, you're aiming to think of a place where you will feel safe, calm and contented. This can be a real place or it can be somewhere you invent. The act of really thinking about what sort of place helps you feel safe can be an important part of preparing to bring the image to life in your imagination in the exercise we're about to do – maybe you've never really have thought about this before. Try to engage in the exercise with curiosity and interest, as if you were an artist designing something for the first time, seeing if you like this here or prefer that there.

If you are using a real place, try not to use one that has other feelings attached. For example, someone I worked with initially wanted to use the bedroom she slept in at her grandparents' house when she was a child. On the face of it this place held good memories of feeling safe and cared for. Sadly, her grandparents had recently passed away, so remembering this room brought back her grief. Instead we built an ideal bedroom as her image; this had some features of her real room, but others that were new enough to help her feel safe.

Some people like to have an actual picture of their safe place and to focus on this while they do the exercise. Other people like to have particular smells or sounds around them that they associate with their safe place. So, for example, one person I worked with liked to have a particular hand cream with her because she associated the smell with her safe place. These kinds of associations can be helpful in activating your soothing system in day-to-day life, as you may be able to keep the sound on your MP3 player or the smell on a handkerchief and use them to rapidly activate your memory of safeness at any time where you feel under threat.

## EXERCISE 5.3: IMAGINING YOUR SAFE PLACE

Begin by finding somewhere comfortable to sit where you will not be disturbed for at least ten minutes. Establish your soothing rhythm breathing.

### Feeling safe

When you feel ready, try to create a place in your mind that could give you the feeling of safeness and calmness. You can close your eyes if you feel OK with this. If you'd rather not, focus your attention on the image in your mind, or on a reminder of your safe place (for example, a particular scent or piece of material, or even a photograph). Alternatively you can focus your attention on your pebble or shell and imagine your safe place, again without closing your eyes.

When you feel you've got some kind of fleeting, impressionistic idea of a safe place, you can start trying to fill out the detail by going through your sensory impressions, starting with the visual ones – for example, what sort of colours are around you? If you're outside, are you on a beach (is it sandy, rocky, pebbly?), in a garden (formal or wild? What kinds of flowers or other plants?) or perhaps in the country (are there trees around? Animals in the fields? Is the sky blue or cloudy, or is the sun rising or setting?)? Then think about any sound you can hear, because sometimes people find sounds create a sense of safeness. One person liked to imagine the sound of a little waterfall. You might hear birdsong, or the crackling of a log fire. Then think of any other sensations, such as a gentle cooling breeze or the warmth of the sun on your face; perhaps the smell of hay, or of a salt breeze on the shore. Going through the sensory details of the image can be quite helpful to fix it and make it real.

Your wandering mind will take you away from this place. So just notice where it goes, and then gently return your attention to the elements of your image that feel safest. When you have the image back, gently expand it again to other parts of your safe place.

Some people find it helpful to imagine seeing themselves in their safe place; to imagine the look on their face, and how they would sit or lie when they were feeling safe, relaxed and contented. Other people don't want to see themselves there, and prefer just to imagine their safe place and their feeling of being in it. It is OK to do either.

There is no 'right or wrong' about your safe place. It is just a place where *you* feel safe. You may find that different images work better at different times of the day, or when you are experiencing different levels or kinds of threat or distress.

After a little practice you may find an image that really works for you. Remember, it is not going to be in complete 'HD 3D surround-sound and smello-vision' – it's an internal image, not a high-tech film – so the more reminders you can develop to help you focus on your image the better. When you have a safe place you find helpful, you can write your own script to help you recall and stay in your safe place. You might even want to record this to make your own CD that you can play back to yourself.

### Feeling wanted

In compassion focused therapy we add an extra important element to our 'safe place' image, which again is designed to stimulate your soothing and compassion systems. After you've been in your safe place for a few minutes and when you're ready, just dwell on the fact that this place is your creation, and therefore really welcomes you and wants you to be here and wants to offer you safeness and rest. The feeling of being wanted by a place may seem strange, but try it and see how you get on. Just focus on feeling that you are in harmony with this place. You might find that if you allow your face to relax into a gentle expression of contentment or compassion, this helps with the experience. At all times remember that nothing is being forced here. You're not trying to *make* yourself feel safe in this image; you are engaging in a gentle, curious practice to see how a sense of safeness might develop over time and how your image might change along with that sense of safeness.

Don't worry if you find yourself feeling quite sleepy when you do this exercise. This is quite common, and some people even use it to help them sleep. That's OK too. However, the main aim is to activate our soothing system, so that we can think about our difficulties a little more easily than we can when we are caught up in the drive or threat system.

## Switching on the compassionate mind

In Chapter 4 we explored how different mindsets can affect our motivations, thoughts, feelings and behaviour. In Chapter 7 we will build upon this idea to help you develop a personal understanding of the different mindsets you experience in relation to food and eating. In this chapter and the next we will work on developing your 'compassion mindset'. The idea is that you will be able to use the skills and attributes of this mindset to help you deal with the experiences that in the past have prompted you to turn to eating – and also to deal with any emotional consequences of giving up overeating.

So a little down the line we're going to be looking at how we can switch from, say, a dieting or a comfort-seeking mindset to a compassionate mindset. But first it's worth looking at how switching mindsets occurs naturally. Let's imagine we are walking down the street planning our next diet. We are likely to be thinking about why we want to diet, the food we need to buy to help us diet, the activities we will start doing to help us lose weight, and all of the good things that will happen for us when we lose weight. We may even start to experience some of the positive feelings we associate with being successful in losing weight. At this point our attention is focused inwards, towards our plans for the future and the positive experiences we expect to get from dieting.

Suddenly we see a small child run out into the road. A car skids to a halt and the child is standing in the middle of the road crying. At this point we will almost certainly find that our attention has instantly switched to the events going on around us. We are focused on the child's distress and rush to help them, perhaps putting an arm round them and helping them to the pavement. We may look around to see if the parent is nearby or, when we feel the child is safe, look after the shocked driver.

Without our making any conscious decision, the event has switched on our compassionate mindset. Our response has been automatic; we haven't decided not to think about our diet any more, we've just forgotten about it as something more important has claimed our attention.

This switch of attention is often associated with a rapid change in our thoughts, feelings and bodily experiences. Witnessing this type of incident can be quite upsetting. Our sympathy for the child, parent and driver may lead to our feeling upset for them. We may find ourselves dwelling on how things could have been far worse, or on the things we wanted to do to help but couldn't do (for example, stopping the child before they ran into the road). We may feel a bit shaky, even tearful. A little later, once the incident is over, we may find that our compassionate mind focuses on other ways we could have helped, or on wondering how the child, parent and driver are. We may find it difficult to think about our diet for the rest of the day while our compassionate mind remains concerned about the people involved in the near-miss. Or we may find that another mindset takes over to help us with the feelings of distress that the incident has called up in us. We may use our comfort-seeking mindset to help us. Alternatively, we may use our dieting mindset to take our thoughts away from the events we have witnessed.

If we could stay with our compassionate mind, but redirect it towards ourselves, we could help ourselves to understand and sympathize with the distress that seeing this incident has caused us. This response is likely to help us manage our feelings better than either the dieting or the comfort-seeking mindset, and to enable us to react in compassionate ways again if we are faced with a similar situation in the future. A compassionate response may congratulate us on our humanity, and value our compassion for others, while at the same time thinking about ways in which we can support ourselves while we're still feeling upset about what we've seen – for example, talking it though with someone else. It may focus on the good we *have* done, rather than on all the things that we *could have* done.

As you can see from the above example, our minds are pretty flexible, with the ability to refocus our attention to help us to manage life's challenges. And as you can also see, our compassionate minds can switch on pretty automatically for other people. However, we can find it a lot harder when it comes to being compassionate with ourselves.

## Exercises to develop the compassionate mind

The compassion focused exercises in this section use imagery and are designed to create the feelings that accompany the experience and practice of compassion, both towards others and towards ourselves. The exercises are adapted from those on the Compassionate Mind Foundation website (for details, see the 'Useful resources' section at the back of this book), with the kind permission of Paul Gilbert and the Foundation. Many people that I have worked with on eating problems find the structure that these exercises offer very helpful. As always in compassion focused therapy, it is important that you work through them at your pace and decide which work best for you.

The compassion focused therapy exercises that follow are focused in four main ways:

- *Developing the inner compassionate self.* In these exercises we will be focusing on creating a sense of a compassionate self, just as actors do if they are trying to get into a role.

- *Compassion flowing out from you to others.* These exercises focus on the feelings in your body when you fill your mind with compassionate feelings for other people.

- *Compassion flowing into you.* Here you will focus on opening up to compassion, to stimulate areas of your brain that are responsive to the kindness of others.

- *Self-compassion.* This set of exercises is focused on developing feelings, thoughts and experiences that direct your capacity for compassion towards yourself. This is just as important as changing your eating patterns: working on the things that can make us overeat can be difficult, and learning how to generate self-compassion can be very helpful during these times, particularly to help us with our emotions.

## Developing the inner compassionate self

As we have seen, we all have the capacity to experience different mindsets and act accordingly. We are men and women of many parts! In the next exercises we will be working to develop the compassionate part of ourselves. We'll begin by taking a look at the key qualities of the compassionate self.

### Wisdom

This has two important aspects. The first is acknowledging that all of us just find ourselves here, with a particular set of genes inherited from our ancestors and a very complicated brain that evolved over many millions of years – neither of which we designed or chose. The second is acknowledging that our sense of self and our memories come from our own experience of life, beginning with the relationships and situations into which we were born.

Our compassionate self knows that we had no choice over the design of our body and brain, or over the life into which we were born. So we further acknowledge that while working with some of what goes on in our minds – powerful emotions, mood shifts, unwanted thoughts or images, and painful memories – can be difficult, there is no point in blaming ourselves for things over which we have had no control. We just found ourselves here, and have to deal with what we find as best we can, using the brain and body we inherited and the experiences of life we gather.

## Strength

This kind of strength is also called fortitude and is related to courage. It is not an aggressive power, but a source of inner confidence and authority that comes from wisdom. Strength helps to maintain our commitment and determination to face and heal suffering.

## Warmth

The compassionate intention to relieve suffering is not cold or clinical but warm, friendly and gentle. The warmth of compassion is not (just) about being nice – it can be firm and persistent – but ensures that all its efforts are made out of a real desire to be helpful and not critical, soothing and not harsh, and are expressed in a gentle, warm, friendly and open voice and manner.

## Responsibility

Compassion is focused on facing rather than turning away from life's challenges. It involves recognizing that even though we didn't cause many of the problems we face, we can still make a commitment to ourselves and others to do something about them, even if we work only in small steps. So assuming responsibility is not about blaming or criticizing, but is about genuinely wanting to act in ways that are helpful and based on our wisdom, strength, warmth and desire to improve things for the future.

It can be helpful to practise focusing on each of these key qualities in turn and imagine having each one, noting what it feels like and any effect this has on your body.

## EXERCISE 5.4: ENVISAGING THE COMPASSIONATE SELF

This exercise is designed to help you focus on the feelings associated with creating compassion in yourself. It is hard to offer ourselves, or others, compassion if we don't have a good idea what this feels like. As you do this exercise and the ones that follow, keep in mind that it doesn't matter whether you feel you have these qualities or not. It is the act of imagining that you have them that is important. This is the kind of approach that 'method' actors use to get into a role: they imagine themselves to have the characteristics of the character they're playing. In this way they are stimulating certain qualities in their minds and bodies, and as a result their acting is convincing, because for the short time when they are 'in character' they in effect 'become' that character. Of course, when they come out of the role they may not want to be anything like the character (particularly if they are playing someone like Hannibal Lecter!), whereas in compassion focused work the idea is that over time you will want to retain the aspects of the role you've been practising: but for the purposes of this exercise it's just putting yourself into that mental state that's important. As with so many exercises, the more you practise this the easier you'll probably find it.

What you will do in this exercise is take each of the qualities we've just described in turn – wisdom, strength, warmth, responsibility; hold it in your mind; and imagine yourself having it. Work through each quality steadily, playfully and slowly. You may find some qualities easier to imagine yourself having than others – and this is perfectly normal. Try to notice how each quality can affect your body differently. Remember that you may get only glimmers of images and feelings, perhaps because your mind wanders or you can't really focus. This is very typical of what happens when we're trying something new, just as if we were trying to learn to play a piano we'd be all fingers and thumbs to start with. Regular practice will help.

So, to begin the exercise, find a place where you can sit quietly and will not be disturbed for at least ten minutes. Establish your soothing breathing rhythm. When you feel that your body has slowed down (even slightly), you are ready to practise imagining that you are a very deeply compassionate person. Think of all the qualities that you would ideally have as that compassionate person. Try to spend at least one minute focusing on each quality – longer if you can.

Now focus on your desire to become a compassionate person and to be able to think, act and feel compassionately. Imagine being a wise person, with a wisdom that comes from your understanding about the nature of our lives, minds and bodies. You are wise enough to know that much of what goes on inside of us is not our fault but the result of our evolution and of experiences over which we had no control.

When you are ready and have a sense of your wisdom, you can switch to imagining having strength, maturity and authority. Explore your body posture (sitting or standing confidently and assertively) and your facial expressions when you are in this mode. Keep your head upright rather than letting it drop forward; your sitting or standing posture should be one of confidence. Remember, you are imagining yourself as a person that understands your own difficulties and those of others in a non-judgemental way, and has the confidence to be sensitive to suffering and to tolerate distress in order to gain better understanding of how to alleviate it.

When you have a sense of your wisdom and strength, you can switch to focusing on qualities of warmth – a gentle friendliness. Imagine being warm and kind. Create a compassionate facial expression. Try to imagine yourself speaking to someone and hear the warm tone of your voice.

Now reach out with that warmth to feel what it might be like to offer it to another.

Next, switch to imagining feelings of responsibility. Imagine that you have lost interest in condemning or blaming and just want to do the best you can to help yourself, and others, move forward. Hold on to your compassionate facial expression and warmth, but focus now on this experience of committing yourself to a compassionate path of self-development.

Finally, you can imagine yourself having all of these qualities and incorporating them into the way you are with yourself and others.

When you have finished, bring yourself gently back into the room. You might want to write down what it felt like to have these qualities and how it might affect the way you want to act in the future.

### EXERCISE 5.5: YOU AT YOUR BEST

Another way you can explore and get close to the idea of your compassionate self is to remind yourself of a time when you felt compassion and/or acted in a compassionate way – it doesn't matter to what degree. When we are struggling with difficult things in our lives it can be easy to forget that we have the capacity for compassion at all, so actively bringing these memories to mind can help you to remember that you do have these qualities within you and to bring them to the fore again. You can think of your compassionate self as 'you at your best'.

It's a good idea to begin by establishing your soothing breathing rhythm, or your safe place image. Then bring to mind a time when you were kind and compassionate to somebody. Choose an occasion when you were satisfied with how helpful you were, and try not to focus on times when you have been compassionate with someone who is very distressed – especially if this is the first time you've tried this exercise. It may help to write down the specific memory you want to focus on, and to 'risk assess' it first, making sure it is not too distressing for you to work with – otherwise you might find yourself focusing on the other person's distress, and maybe your inability entirely to alleviate it, rather than bringing your attention to your own compassionate qualities. The aim is to focus on your feelings of wanting to help and your kindness.

So, once you have brought to mind an appropriate occasion, focus on how you felt as a result of being kind and compassionate. As you develop your image of 'you at your best', focus on your body position, facial expression and tone of voice as you offer your wisdom, strength, warmth and courage. Spend sufficient time on this exercise to really be able to explore it thoroughly and reflect on the experience.

Both these exercises draw on Buddhist ideas to do with developing key qualities of the self (such as mindfulness and compassion), which in turn give us new insights into the nature of the self. When we see the compassionate self as the self we would like to become, in a way this is no different from wanting to develop any other aspect of the self. If we want to be good at sport, an accomplished pianist, a good cook or well read in poetry – we know that we would need to practise. The more we practise, the closer we get to being what we want to become. Some days our practice won't go very well, but this doesn't mean that over the long term we can't move towards our goal of becoming the kind of person – sportsperson, pianist, cook or literary scholar – we would like to be.

It's exactly the same with the self. We can make a decision to become more like the compassionate self of our imagination. We can practise what we would like to become by imagining, enacting, thinking and playing with those compassionate qualities. If we have an argument with somebody, we can reflect with the compassionate self on how we might deal with that situation better in the future. If we have problems with food, we can learn to be compassionate rather than angry and critical, and gently and kindly think about how to help ourselves next time. There is nothing fixed about our personality – we can make choices about it, and with practice can move closer to the kind of person we want to be.

## Compassion every day

Ideally, try to practise 'becoming the compassionate self' each day. As well as doing the exercises when you have time, you can also fit practice into even the smallest slots in a busy life. When you wake up in the morning, try to spend a few minutes practising becoming your compassionate self. As you lie in bed, bring a compassionate expression to your face and focus on your real desire to be wise and compassionate. Remember, inside you, you have the capacity for wisdom and strength – but you have to create space for it. If you practise for even two minutes a day, every day, it is likely to have an effect. You can also practise while you're standing at the bus stop or lying in the bath. You may then find you'll want to practise for longer periods of time and perhaps to make more time during your day for this. Meanwhile, whenever you are aware of the opportunity, even sitting in a meeting, you can use soothing breathing and focus on becoming the wise, compassionate, calm, mature self.

## Compassion flowing out from you to others

The idea of the next three exercises is to focus on the desire to help and on feelings of kindness and warmth. If the feelings don't come easily, don't worry; it is your behaviour and intentions that are important – the feelings may follow on behind. In the first of this group of exercises we simply get into our compassionate mindset and imagine our compassion flowing into someone we care about, giving them three key compassionate messages. In the second you will be focusing your compassion on helping a particular individual you care about who is struggling with something in their lives and whom you would like to support using your compassionate self.

The final exercise in this group can be a little trickier for some people. Many people who overeat are actually critical of others who overeat and find it difficult to be compassionate with them. In a way they can be a reflection of ourselves and our own struggles – and, if we are very critical of ourselves, we can also be very critical of what we see in the mirror! One way to overcome this obstacle is to personalize things; it can be far harder to be uncompassionate with a specific person than with an idea or abstract group of people. Exercise 5.8 builds on your innate wisdom and compassion for others by directly focusing your attention on offering compassion to people who overeat.

Of course, many people who overeat are very sympathetic with the struggles of others, but find it difficult to offer themselves the same level of compassion. Indeed, I find this all the time in the groups I run. Exercise 5.8 is the beginning of offering yourself compassion for your difficulties with overeating – but please only try to work on it when you feel that you can do Exercises 5.6 and 5.7 quite comfortably and are starting to feel your compassionate emotions coming into action – even if only a little.

### Exercise 5.6: Focusing compassion on others

First find a time and place when you can sit quietly without being disturbed for at least ten minutes. Now try to create a sense of being a compassionate person as best you can, as you did in Exercise 5.4. Some days this will be easier than others – even just the slightest glimmer can be a start. Now bring to mind someone you care about: this might be your partner, a friend, parent or child, or a pet or other animal. When you have this individual in mind, focus on directing towards them three basic thoughts (if you're familiar with Buddhism, you may recognize this traditional text or mantra):

*May you be well.*
*May you be happy.*
*May you be free of suffering.*

Keep in mind that it is your behaviour and intentions that are important – the feelings may follow on behind. Be gentle, take time, and allow yourself to focus on desires and wishes you create in yourself for the other person or animal. Maybe picture them smiling or looking affectionately at you and being happy to receive your compassionate wishes. Spend time focusing on this genuine desire of yours for the well-being of another individual.

Do this exercise mindfully: that is, if your mind wanders, that's not a problem – just gently and kindly bring it back to the task. Try to notice any physical or emotional feelings that emerge from this exercise. Don't worry if nothing much happens at a conscious level; the act of having a go is the important thing. It's like getting fit – it may take several visits to the gym or training sessions before you consciously notice feeling different, but your body will be responding straight away.

### Exercise 5.7: Compassion flowing out to others in difficulty

In this exercise we are again going to imagine kindness and compassion flowing from you out to another person or animal, but in this case that other individual will be facing a difficulty that you want to help them with. As with Exercise 5.5, try not to choose a time when that person (or animal) was very distressed, because then you are likely to focus on the distress, and possibly your inability to dispel it, rather than on your own compassionate feelings. It can help to prepare by jotting down the name of the person or animal you want to help, and the difficulty you want to help them with. Before you start, try to make sure that the issue will not be so distressing for you that you cannot do the exercise.

Begin by establishing your soothing breathing rhythm or your safe place as a basis for your compassionate mindset. Now move into the following sequence of stages, trying to spend at least one minute on each element of the exercise.

(1) When you feel ready, bring to mind a time when you felt compassionate towards the person or animal you have in mind.

(2) Imagine yourself expanding, as if you are becoming calmer, wiser, stronger and more mature, and better able to help that individual. Pay attention to your body as you remember your feelings of kindness.

(3) Now imagine warmth spreading within your body and flowing over the other person or animal. Feel your genuine desire for this other individual to be free of suffering and to flourish.

(4) Now focus on your tone of voice and the kinds of things you would want to say or do to help them.

(5) Next think about your pleasure in being able to be kind.

(6) To finish, focus on combining all of these qualities in your compassionate self and imagine them flowing into the other person or animal: your desire to be helpful and kind; feelings of expansion; the sense of warmth; your tone of voice; the wisdom in your voice and in your behaviour.

When you have finished the exercise, you might want to make some notes about how doing this exercise made you feel.

## EXERCISE 5.8: COMPASSION FOR PEOPLE WHO OVEREAT

There are several ways to do this exercise. The first step is to identify the person or people that you want your compassion to flow towards. Some people find it easier to offer their compassion to someone they know personally who overeats; other people find it easier to offer compassion to someone they don't know personally (for example, someone from a TV dieting programme, or someone they've seen in a newspaper); other people find it easier to offer it to everyone who struggles with overeating. For the purposes of the exercise it really doesn't matter which you choose. The key point here is to learn to feel compassion for people who struggle with overeating.

Then, having identified the person or people you want to offer compassion to, decide whether you would find it easier to offer them general compassion (Exercise 5.6) or compassion for a specific difficulty (Exercise 5.7) before you move on to offering them compassion for the struggles they may have with their eating. Start with the exercises you find easier, and then build towards the practice you find more difficult.

So this is how you do it. Find a place to sit comfortably and then establish your soothing breathing rhythm, or your safe place image. When you feel ready, imagine becoming a compassionate person – you at your best. Remember to keep a confident posture and an upright stance. Go through the key qualities of compassion in a secure and wise person, believing yourself to be strong, confident and deeply kind. You realize how difficult life is because of the brain that we have evolved with.

Now in your mind's eye see somebody who overeats. Watch them. Understand that the motives and desires causing them to overeat are complex and can often cause them distress. You may also focus your compassion on the unintended consequences that overeating can have for them. Using your wisdom, recognize how they're caught up in a pattern of feelings and behaviour that they didn't design and probably don't want. You're not trying to change anything about them at this point – just learning to be compassionate for them and to them. Imagine them getting as much compassion as they need. For example, you may see yourself alongside them and saying, 'You're going through a tough time at the moment,' 'I can see how hard this is for you,' or 'I can see that food is a real comfort for you,' or trying to help them find ways to help them manage the problems that cause them to overeat.

Give yourself plenty of time to just keep your compassionate mind gently focused on what you're seeing in front of you. As you do this, you may begin to have feelings about what would be helpful to the person you're watching. However, if you feel your mind becoming angry, critical or irritated with them then break the image, pull back and refocus on the soothing, rhythmical breathing or safe place until you notice these feelings ease a little; then re-engage with your compassionate self before recommencing the imagery. It is not unusual to have only fleeting feelings of compassion for people who overeat, and you may need to gently redirect your compassion for them several times during the exercise.

When you have finished, bring yourself gently back into the room, and note down how you feel now, and how you might act differently towards people who overeat from a more compassionate perspective. You might also want to reflect on your experience from your own perspective. What came up for you? Was there anything that surprised you? What would you like to work on to improve your capacity to respond to overeating with compassion?

## Compassion flowing into you

Although many of us can see how being offered, and being able to accept, compassion can be helpful for other people, we can find it quite difficult to accept for ourselves. Our compassionate mind has the capacity both to give compassion to others and to receive it from them. As we have seen, our capacity to receive compassion is crucial to activating our soothing system, and hence to helping us manage difficult events and emotions. In the next two exercises we will practise allowing compassion from others into our lives. The first exercise is focused on helping us to remember times when other people have offered us compassion. When we are distressed, our threat system naturally focuses on things that are dangerous to us, and this may mean that we temporarily forget that some people in the world have been compassionate to us. The key here is to nurture those memories and use them as a basis for helping us to engage with those in our lives who can be compassionate, to recognize compassion when it is offered and to use it to help us.

Sadly, sometimes people cannot remember other people being particularly compassionate towards them. This can be for a variety of reasons. Perhaps they are so distressed that it is hard to bring back any memory of kindness; or maybe they have just not had very many experiences of other people being compassionate towards them. Sometimes people struggle to recall these memories because the compassion they were offered was conditional, with a price tag that they don't want to remember. For example, they might have been offered compassion at one moment and hostility the next from someone very unpredictable. Sometimes, too, memories of compassion from another are too painful to bring to mind because the person is no longer around.

So it's not always easy to find a memory of being offered compassion. If your experiences make this difficult for you, for one reason or another, that's sad, but it's not something you can blame yourself for, nor is it a sign of any failure or personal inadequacy on your part. It is simply the way it is! It does, however, create a practical problem in that it means you will need to build up from scratch an image of compassion flowing into you from others. The second exercise in this section is designed to address this need by developing an image of someone or something that can offer us compassion throughout our lives, a compassionate companion we can always rely on. It is possible to do this even if you have limited experience of compassion from others by drawing on your innate wisdom about compassion that you have used in Exercise 5.5 ('you at your best').

EXERCISE 5.9: COMPASSION FLOWING INTO YOU: USING YOUR MEMORIES

This exercise asks you to recall a memory of someone being compassionate towards you. This memory shouldn't be of a time when you were very distressed, because you will then focus on the distress rather than the compassion: the point of the exercise is to focus on the desire of another person to help and be kind to you. Try to spend a minute or so on each phase of the exercise.

To begin, engage in your soothing breathing rhythm for a minute or so until you can feel your body slowing down.

(1) When you feel ready, bring to mind a memory of a time when someone was kind to you.

(2) Allow your face to relax into a compassionate expression and your body to adopt a posture which gives you a sense of kindness and a warm glow or feeling of gratitude as you recall the memory.

(3) Explore the facial expressions and body position of the person who was kind to you. Sometimes it helps if you see them moving towards you, or see their face breaking into a smile, or their head on one side.

(4) Now focus on the important sensory qualities of your memory. First spend just one minute focusing on the kinds of things this person said and the tone of their voice. Then focus on the emotion in the person, what they really felt for you at that moment.

(5) Now focus on the whole experience, maybe whether they held you, touched you, offered you a tissue or helped you in other ways. Notice how they created a feeling of being soothed and connected in you, and your sense of gratitude and pleasure at being helped. Allow the experience of soothing, connectedness, gratitude and joy in being helped to grow. Remember to keep your facial expression as compassionate as you can.

When you are ready, gently let the memory fade, come out of the exercise and make some notes on how you felt. You may notice that bringing these memories to mind has created feelings inside you, even if they are just glimmers. What came up for you? Was there anything that surprised you? What would you like to work on to improve your capacity to receive compassion from others?

## Inventing the 'compassionate other'

When we experience compassion and kindness from another person, when we feel and sense that another mind is focused on us with benevolence, it can have quite a powerful impact on us. Our brains have evolved to be very responsive to receiving kindness from others. We want to develop exercises that will help trigger those responses, because in doing so we create a sense of being soothed and also an inner security. So how do we do this if we can't recall any real experiences of receiving compassion? We practise using an idea of a 'compassionate other' whom we create for ourselves. Some people say, 'Well, it's all very well imagining compassionate others, but I want real ones in my life.' Of course, we all want compassionate relationships with other people. These exercises are not meant to replace real relationships. They are designed to stimulate your brain to help you with your feelings and emotions. Developing these aspects of our brain can also help us to feel safe enough to create and foster compassionate relationships with other people in the outside world. So it is not a matter of either/or. If I can use a sporting analogy again, practising in the gym is not the same as playing the real game. But it can help us when we do play the game for real.

### EXERCISE 5.10: CREATING A COMPASSIONATE COMPANION

In this exercise we're going to create your 'ideal compassionate other'. If you could imagine or create a being that would encapsulate everything you could possibly desire from someone totally focused on your welfare – what kind of qualities would they have?

Now, some people may of course dismiss this idea straight away with thoughts like 'I don't deserve that' or 'If anybody got really close to me and knew me from the inside they wouldn't like me.' However, for the purposes of this exercise this is all beside the point, which is *to imagine* that you are the recipient of complete compassion from another mind without judgement in the present moment.

Whatever image comes to mind or you choose to work with, it is *your* creation and therefore your own personal ideal of who or what you would most like to care for and about you. It is not uncommon for people to choose an inanimate object (like a tree or a colour). Some people prefer their image to be that of an animal or a fantasy character (like a dog or fairy). Some people can bring to mind a fictional character from a book or film (e.g. Gandalf from *The Lord of the Rings*), while some prefer to invent their own individual person or creature. You can choose a real person you actually know, although in my experience this can be a little tricky. Most people we know are not compassionate all the time – after all, they are only human, like us! Also, it's very tempting to choose someone who has been very caring but may no longer be with us – perhaps a teacher, friend or relative who may have passed away or moved on and whom we no longer see. Thus our image can get mixed up with feelings of grief and longing, which can distract us from the aim of this exercise, which is to experience receiving compassion from our ideal compassionate other.

Whatever your companion looks like, it is important that you give them certain qualities. These include the key qualities of the compassionate self that we identified earlier in this chapter, and are present in complete and perfect form in the ideal compassionate other:

- a deep commitment to you: a desire to help you cope with and relieve your suffering, and take joy in your happiness;

- strength of mind that is not overwhelmed by your pain or distress, but remains present, enduring it with you;

- wisdom that has been gained through experience and truly understands the struggles you go through in life;

- warmth, conveyed by kindness, gentleness, caring and openness;

- an acceptance that is never judgemental or critical but understands your struggles and accepts you as you are, while also being deeply committed to helping and supporting you.

You can use Worksheet 1 ('Building your compassionate companion') to help you with this exercise. The key is to focus on the feelings, and on the experience of imagining another mind that fervently wants you to flourish. When you have completed the worksheet you are ready to begin the imagery part of the exercise.

Sitting in a place where you won't be disturbed, first establish your soothing breathing rhythm and allow your face to relax into a compassionate expression. Then bring to mind your safe place. This may now be the place where you wish to create and meet your compassionate image – or you can choose to meet your compassionate companion in another place; that's OK too. The key thing is to create the feelings of being safe and soothed before you meet your compassionate companion.

Now imagine your compassionate companion appearing in your safe place; they may be materializing from the mist, walking in though a door, or appearing in some other way. Imagine them sitting or standing beside you. You may want to touch them or be held by them, and that's OK, but only allow your compassionate companion to be with you in a way you feel comfortable with and that helps you to feel safe and soothed.

To begin with, simply practise experiencing what it is like to focus on the feeling that another mind really values you and cares about you unconditionally. Now focus on your compassionate companion and imagine they are looking at you with great warmth. Imagine that they have the following desires for you:

> *That you be well.*
> *That you be happy.*
> *That you be free of suffering.*

Try to allow yourself to open up to the experiences of compassion, in the knowledge that you can always rely on your compassionate companion to offer you their commitment to you, their strength, wisdom and acceptance.

You may notice that your mind wanders, perhaps to memories of times when people have not been compassionate towards you. This is perfectly normal. Just gently bring your mind back to the task in hand, which is focusing your attention on experiencing compassion from your companion.

Try to do this exercise for about ten minutes; then gently bring yourself back into the here and now and jot down in your notebook what you felt during the exercise.

## Struggling with the idea of a compassionate companion

It is common for people to struggle to develop this image of an ideal compassionate other. For example, you might have thought, 'Yes, but this is not real, I want somebody real to care for me.' That is, of course, very

### Worksheet 1: Building your compassionate companion

| |
|---|
| How would you like your ideal caring, compassionate image to look/appear? What are its visual qualities? |
| How would you like your ideal caring, compassionate image to sound, e.g. tone of voice? |
| What other sensory qualities can you give to it, e.g. its smell or textures? |
| How would you like your ideal caring, compassionate image to relate to you? (For example: in a caring, warm, understanding way) |
| How would you like to relate to your ideal caring, compassionate image? (For example: allowing it to care for you, listening to its wisdom and concern for you) |

understandable. It's even possible that doing this exercise could make you feel sad, because we all have an innate desire for genuine connection with others. However, as I pointed out in the introduction to this exercise, in a way these reservations are missing the point of the exercise. Of course it is desirable to find people who care for us and to be able to accept their compassion. But sometimes, though we have these people in our lives, we can't allow their compassion in because we haven't learned how to accept it. And at other times we could accept compassion but just don't have such people available to us.

The aim here is to help you develop the compassionate aspect of yourself that you may already be able to direct towards other people, but may struggle to direct towards yourself. Your ideal compassionate companion allows you to practise receiving compassion at a pace and in a way that feels safe for you, and from a source that is available to you whenever you need it.

## Self-compassion

This may be the hardest of all of the exercises we have introduced so far. Many of us struggle to be compassionate towards ourselves. We will take a closer look at why this may be in the next chapter. For now, you are simply going to try to practise directing compassion towards yourself using the skills you have learned in the exercises you have already done.

In these previous exercises you have practised offering compassion to a person, or people, who overeat. You may have found this tricky. If you are very critical of your own eating habits, this is probably not the best place to begin your journey to becoming self-compassionate. Instead, you may want to offer yourself compassion for other difficulties in your life – perhaps the things that trigger your overeating.

Sometimes people find it difficult to jump straight into offering themselves compassion. This is where your compassionate companion can be really helpful. You can imagine them feeling compassion for you relating to another difficulty you have experienced, such as a loss or a health problem – ideally one that is not overwhelmingly distressing, otherwise you might get caught up in the distress rather than the feeling of compassion. As you become more confident in using your compassionate companion to support you, you can always increase the difficulty of the problems or situations that you bring to them.

Of course, we know that your compassionate companion is not real: it simply represents the kindest, strongest, wisest and warmest parts of you. However, it can be a useful bridge until you are able to offer yourself compassion directly. Try the exercise below to get you started.

EXERCISE 5.11: USING YOUR COMPASSIONATE COMPANION TO HELP YOU

Find a time and place when you can sit quietly without being disturbed. Now establish your soothing breathing rhythm and allow your face to relax into its compassionate expression. Then bring to mind the safe place where you want to meet your companion. At this point you are ready to begin the exercise: try to spend at least one minute on each element.

(1) First, imagine spending some time with your companion and experiencing their compassion flowing over and around you. You may want to touch them or be held by them; this is fine, but remember only to allow your compassionate companion to be with you in a way you feel comfortable with and that helps you to feel safe and soothed.

(2) Next, focus on your compassionate companion looking at you with great warmth. Imagine that they have the following wishes and hopes for you:

> *That you be well.*
> *That you be happy.*
> *That you be free of suffering.*

(3) Allow yourself to sit with and open up to these experiences of compassion, in the knowledge that you can always rely on your compassionate companion to offer you their commitment to you, their strength, wisdom and acceptance.

(4) Next, imagine telling your compassionate companion about the struggle that you are having. Imagine their facial expression and body posture as they listen to you with concern and acceptance.

(5) If you can, imagine what they would say to you to help you have the courage, wisdom and strength to face your difficulty. Perhaps they will come up with other ways of seeing things, or suggest other ways to help you. Perhaps they cannot. It doesn't really matter – what is important is that you experience their warmth and kindness, strength and wisdom, and that you feel you can express the worries or feelings that are troubling you without being judged or criticized.

(6) Draw the exercise to a close by once more experiencing the compassion flowing from your companion into you. Allow yourself to take pleasure in the feelings of safeness, comfort and connectedness for a while before you gently bring yourself back into the room.

You may want to note down how you felt about this experience, and any new understandings or ways of coping that you have learned from your companion.

### Exercise 5.12: Being the focus of self-compassion

This exercise is similar to Exercise 5.6 on page 115. The only difference is that you are focusing your compassionate attention on yourself, rather than on someone else.

Find a time and place when you can sit quietly without being disturbed. Now try to create a sense within yourself of being a compassionate person. When you can do this, bring to mind a picture of yourself. Sometimes it can help to use a photograph or look at your face in the mirror. If you have a strong sense of self-dislike or self-criticism for the way you are now, it may be helpful to use an image of you as a child.

When you have an image in your mind, focus on directing towards yourself the same three basic feelings and thoughts:

*May I be well.*
*May I be happy.*
*May I be free of suffering.*

Keep in mind that it is your behaviour and intentions that are important – the feelings may follow on behind. Maybe you can picture the image of you smiling at back at your compassionate self and feeling joy and gratitude.

As with the other exercises, try this for a couple of minutes at first, then gradually build up to about ten minutes when you feel ready. Your wandering mind is likely to be very active during this exercise, particularly at first. This is quite normal: just gently and kindly bring it back to the task.

When you have finished, note down any thoughts or feelings that emerged while you were doing the exercise, or after you had done it, that you might want to take away from it.

### EXERCISE 5.13: FOCUSING SELF-COMPASSION ON A SPECIFIC PROBLEM

This is the final exercise, and is the most advanced so far in terms of self-compassion. It is a variation on Exercises 5.7 and 5.11. In this case you are practising offering yourself compassion for a specific dilemma or difficulty in your life. As with Exercise 5.11, try to resist the temptation to choose something that is very painful for you at the moment. You can work your way up to this as you grow in confidence with the exercise.

In this exercise we are going to imagine kindness and compassion flowing from you towards yourself. It can help to prepare by jotting down the issue you want to work on. You may also want to use the photograph you used for Exercise 5.12, or to look in the mirror as you do the exercise. Try to spend at least one minute on each element of the exercise.

Begin by establishing your soothing breathing rhythm or your safe place.

(1) When you feel ready, bring to mind your compassionate self. Imagine yourself expanding as if you are becoming calmer, wiser, stronger and more mature, and able to help.

(2) Pay attention to your body as you remember your feelings of kindness.

(3) Now imagine expanding the warmth within your body and imagine it flowing over and around you. Feel your genuine desire for you to be free of suffering and to flourish.

(4) Now focus on your tone of voice and the kind of things you would want to say or do to help you with the problem you are facing. If it helps, you can imagine having a conversation with yourself.

(5) Next think about your pleasure in being able to be kind to yourself and to accept your own kindness.

(6) To finish, focus on combining all these qualities of your compassionate self – the calmness, wisdom, strength and maturity; the warmth, kindness and genuine desire to help – in both voice and behaviour, and imagine them flowing into you.

When you have finished the exercise you might want to make some notes about how it felt for you and what you want to take away from it.

---

### SUMMARY

The exercises set out in this chapter are designed to help you to develop and foster your capacity for compassion, and to learn to direct your compassionate attention towards yourself and others. You may find that they take some effort at first, and you may well find that you do not actually *feel* compassionate, particularly towards yourself, for some time; however, it is crucial that you can at least *act* from a compassionate mindset before you move on to trying to address your overeating. This is why I say in the exercises that it is important to focus on your intentions and behaviour, and that the feelings can follow on behind. It's quite normal to find genuine feelings of compassion hard to generate, especially if you haven't had much experience of compassion from others, or if you have learned to be self-critical. Eventually, though, these feelings do emerge – usually for other people or things before ourselves. It is also normal for these feelings to come and go, particularly when we are distressed. The key is to continue to practise the exercises to gradually build up the habit of compassion, like a 'mental muscle'; as you do so, your brain will gradually change to improve your capacity to give and receive compassion.

It is possible that these exercises may arouse strong feelings or memories. This too is not uncommon, and the important thing is to accept these feelings or recollections with compassion as part of you that may need to be cared for.

In the next chapter we will explore how you can use the habits of compassion that you have learned to help you manage your emotions, including the more difficult ones, and to find ways to face life's challenges without using food as a source of comfort or solace.

# 6 Developing the skills of self-compassion

In the previous chapter we explored ways to work on developing compassionate attention, thinking, feeling and behaviour, both towards others and towards ourselves. This chapter builds on that work in exploring how to use our compassionate focus in a range of practical ways to help us cope with difficult emotions and thoughts – especially those related to eating.

## Managing distress compassionately

Many people find that they eat more when they are distressed, and that doing this helps them to manage their emotions – anger, pain, sadness, guilt, shame, fear, etc. Eating can indeed offer some respite from our immediate emotional distress; however, the relief is usually short-lived because the underlying issues or causes have not been addressed or resolved. Now, sometimes the things that have been causing us distress resolve themselves – but even if they do, if we haven't explicitly addressed them and so don't know *how* they have been resolved, the chances are that next time we are in distress we will turn to food again for the same immediate relief, rather than tolerating the distressing feelings for long enough to investigate them and work out where their real origins lie so that we can deal with them once and for all.

You might ask at this point: Well, if eating works for me every time, why bother to work out what's going on underneath? Sadly, these overeating 'solutions' are not cost-free; they can often lead to cycles of distress and potential health problems. An example of how this pattern can get established is shown in Figure 6.1. Of course, it is perfectly understandable that we do our best to manage unpleasant feelings in any way we can, and in the next three chapters we will explore how overeating, often along with a dieting mindset, has developed to help you do this. So we need to take a compassionate view of these ways of managing distress, not beat

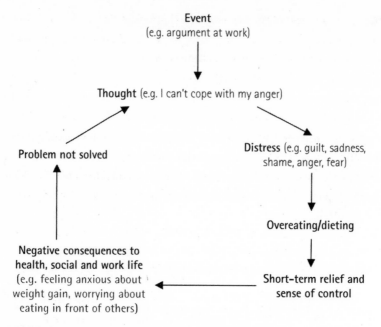

**Figure 6.1:** The vicious circle of distress and overeating

ourselves up for having used them. After all, until we have other ways to manage that we can really rely on, we would be very unwise to give up something we know works, even if it only works temporarily.

It is also helpful to remember that, as we saw in Chapters 2 and 3, our bodies do actually respond to overeating in a way that can help us to feel better – and indeed that the food industry has made the most of this fact. So we're up against both evolution and big business! In exploring alternative ways to manage our feelings, we will look at both short-term solutions, for those times when our feelings are very intense, and also longer-term solutions, in the form of ways to activate our soothing system and work on our feelings and desires without using food.

## Learning to activate our affiliative soothing/ contentment system

As we saw in Chapter 3, our emotional system for soothing and contentment has evolved to help us manage distress by seeking out and using support from others. When we are very distressed this system can become overwhelmed and we will use other ways to manage threats that we experience or feel. We live in a world that can be very stressful, and where there can be very little space for us to experience soothing – or even acknowledgement that we might need it. Indeed, our culture often drives us to associate feeling contented with stimulation: buying new things, eating more food or seeking out new thrills and excitement – buzzes linked to the achievement/drive system in our brain. Sadly, we have lost touch with our need to keep our emotional systems in balance, and the skills of dealing with stress by calming our minds have been sorely neglected.

Imagine your mind as a hot-water boiler. Boilers have a thermostat that switches off the heat when the water is hot enough. Without a thermostat the water just keeps getting hotter and hotter until the boiler explodes. Our emotional regulation systems are a little like this: we have different ways of reducing the pressure. One is 'letting off steam' by distraction, excitement – or eating; another is turning our boiler down by using our soothing system.

A little later in this chapter we will consider why we should learn to tolerate our emotions when they are very 'hot', and how we can do this. However, this takes confidence that we can manage our feelings, and developing the skills of self-soothing is a very important step towards learning to do this. So in this section of the chapter we will first explore how we can lower our overall 'emotional temperature' by turning on our soothing system.

In the previous chapter we learned ways to bring our soothing system into action using our imagination. We will now explore how to use the things we can physically sense around us to do the same thing. We will go through various techniques; the key is to find the ones that help you.

Learning to use our senses of sight, hearing, smell and touch, and mindfully focusing on our sensory experiences, can help us to activate our soothing system. Indeed, some therapy programmes use the experience of nature walks specifically to do this. Here we are trying to immerse ourselves in a sensory experience that helps us to feel calm and contented in a way that feels safe for us. It is likely that you will find that some sensory experiences do this better for you than others. Sometimes the experiences we focus on in our safe place can give us clues to what works best for us. Play with all of your senses to find which ones soothe you. You may well find that different sensory experiences affect you more strongly at different times; this is perfectly normal.

In the following exercises we will explore how to use our senses of sight, hearing, touch and smell to activate our soothing system. Taste can also be a powerful way to bring our soothing system into play; however, as we are trying to break the association between eating and feeling soothed, it is more helpful to avoid this sense as a way to soothe yourself, at least until you are sure that it won't lead to overeating.

## Using our senses to activate our soothing system

### Soothing by sight

Sight – the things we see – can be very powerful in triggering our soothing system. As with all the senses, to find out whether this works for you, the important thing is to try to immerse yourself in the experience; to pay mindful attention to the things you can see.

In choosing what you find soothing to look at, take care to avoid anything that is associated with unpleasant memories or events. People I have worked with have found it soothing to look at a beautiful flower, a lit candle or a burning fire, an intricate shell or a smooth pebble. Alternatively, you may find it more soothing to look at a wider range of things, in which case you may want to visit a museum or gallery; sit in the lobby of a beautiful hotel, take a walk and look at nature around you, or go out in the middle of the night and watch the stars. Some people prefer to make their own scrapbook, or even to make one space in a room visually appealing so they can control the range of things they want to look at.

Whatever you choose, it is likely that your mind will wander when you look at things you find soothing. Again, as with the breathing and safe place exercises, you are not *forcing* yourself to concentrate. Rather, just notice where your mind wanders to and gently return to the visual experience that you find soothing. As with all of these exercises, the more we practise the better we become at using our senses to soothe us. Some days we will find it easier than others to use our senses to soothe us; it can be particularly difficult if we are already close to 'boiling over'.

## Soothing by hearing

We know that humans can be very sensitive to sound. Babies in the womb can be calmed by certain types of music or startled by loud noises. Again, the key is to find the sounds that you find soothing. You may be drawn to beautiful or soothing music – but again, we may need to be a little careful in what music we choose. Musicians throughout the ages have used music to create certain moods in us; so as the idea here is to call up a feeling of being soothed, it's probably best to avoid loud, invigorating or sad music! Some people find the sounds of nature (waves, birds, rainfall or leaves rustling, for example) to be soothing. I personally find some voices soothing and comforting; you may find that a particular actor's voice does this for you, or it may be the voice of someone you know personally. Some people I know use audio books to help soothe them; some even request my voice on a CD to talk them through settling into their safe place.

## Soothing by smell

The fastest way to a man (or woman's) heart – actually, their brain – is not through their stomach, as the popular saying has it; it is through their nose! Our sense of smell is our fastest-acting sensory system – which makes sense in evolutionary terms, as we can often smell danger long before we can see it or hear it, let alone touch it. You may have tried to incorporate smells in your 'safe place' and 'compassionate companion' exercises. If not, this can be a good opportunity to try to find out what smells you find soothing. You could use your favourite perfume or lotions. To save money you can try them at the perfume counter first! You might find that natural smells are more soothing: you can experiment with the smells of different flowers, fruits or other natural products (like pine).

## Soothing by touch

Touch can be a powerful source of soothing. Studies of infant monkeys found that if they were fed without comforting touching, they suffered serious difficulties in their development and grew up to be fearful. There is now a lot of evidence that affectionate touch has many positive effects on us. When we're anxious, being touched by another person who we feel cares for us can reduce our anxiety more quickly than even the most powerful anti-anxiety drugs. This is probably not news to you; it comes to us automatically to reach out and hold our children, friends or partners if they are in distress. The key here is to allow ourselves the opportunity to experience touch in a way that feels safe for us. This can include planning more hugs into your day or having a massage. Even if other people are not around, we can massage ourselves, or even imagine being held (for example by your compassionate companion).

Human touch is not the only tactile experience that can soothe us. Pets can have a similar effect; indeed, some hospital wards even have a 'visiting pet' system because stroking a pet can help soothe clients and even speed up the healing process. Even something that simulates the feel of a pet (for example, a fur-covered hot-water bottle) can be soothing for some of us.

Other tactile experiences that we may find soothing include smoothing a creamy lotion on our hands or body; placing a cold compress on our forehead; or even brushing our hair for a long time. Physical warmth can also be soothing – for example, having a pleasantly warm bath, sunbathing (don't overdo this, though, and make sure to put on some suncream!) or cuddling a hot-water bottle. For other people the experience of slipping into fresh, clean sheets or silky clothes, or sitting back into a comfortable chair, can be very soothing.

You may find that you prefer to be soothed by just one of your senses, or by a combination. The key is to be mindful of the experience and to allow yourself to take joy and pleasure from the experience of being physically soothed. Some people prefer to take a more active approach to being physically soothed, for example taking part in formal relaxation training or meditation classes. Again, this is absolutely fine, as long as you find it activates your soothing system. Remember that your wandering mind may pull you away from any of these experiences, and that you may need to gently refocus on the experience of being soothed.

Aim to practise your physical self-soothing skills every day. You may wish to draw up a list of the types of things you can try, and to practise each one for several days before moving on to try another. Over time you will find your own menu of things you find physically soothing. Sometimes you can get the best of both worlds by practising your physical self-soothing and then moving into your compassion exercises.

## Strategies for coping with a crisis

Practising soothing skills is not a way to stop bad things happening or stop us feeling the ups and downs of life. No matter how good we have become at self-soothing, we are all bound at some time to experience events, emotions or memories that we find difficult to deal with. When this happens it is easy to fall back on unhealthy eating or overeating or dieting to get us through: so what we need are other compassion-focused ways of riding these waves of difficult emotions and situations. There are basically two ways of doing this: one is to try to *distract* yourself from the emotional distress you are experiencing; the other is to learn to compassionately *tolerate* that distress.

So let's explore some techniques you can use to help you distract yourself from your distress or to tolerate it, and thus enable you to cope in new ways with the ups and downs and crises of life. It's important to note that these skills are not about resolving the difficulty underlying your distress, but are designed to help you to cope with it and to support you while you try to deal with the underlying issue – that is, to give you some space for what may be a longer-term task. These are skills for handling painful events and emotions, accepting life as it is at that moment, when we cannot make things better right away.

In the longer term it is more helpful to learn how to tolerate distress for at least long enough to understand what is causing it, and we explore how you can do this a little later in the chapter. However, this skill can take some time to develop, and even then we may still want to have confidence in our ability to manage our distress without using food.

## Distraction techniques

Sometimes we can get as far as deciding that we are not going to use old coping behaviours (such as overeating) but do not feel that we have got to the stage where we can tolerate our distress or rely on new ways of coping. At these times, distracting ourselves from our distress can be very helpful. Distractions – which can be practical, mental and/or emotional – can be a great way of 'buying time' to allow our impulses to subside (for example, the impulse to have an extra biscuit as a treat) and help us realize that we have more control over our impulses than we thought we had.

### Practical distractions

Specific practical activities can include hobbies (e.g. knitting, craft work, painting) or sporting activities; going to social or cultural events; calling or visiting a friend; doing computer games; going for a walk; doing paid or voluntary work; reading; doing puzzles; gardening – even housework! It can be helpful to make a list of all the activities you could use as distractions before you actually need them.

Of course, our minds will still tend to wander, and some things can be more absorbing than others. Some activities, too, have an inbuilt limited time-span – for example, a film on DVD comes to an end – and we may need to plan a variety of activities so that there is always something else we can do. It can also be very easy to take some distractions to extremes (for example, overworking or exercising excessively). So it is also important not to let any distraction become too much of a habit, or to get too far drawn into something that we cannot afford to do, because of either the time it takes or the money it costs us. Remember, this is simply a short-term way to help you cope.

Practical activities that help other people as well can have the double benefit of providing a useful distraction and also helping to activate our compassionate mind. Examples of these include volunteer work; giving something to someone else; making something nice for another person; or planning and doing a surprising, thoughtful thing for someone that you know they will like.

Simple physical sensations can be helpful as a very short-term distraction – for example, holding something cold, squeezing a rubber ball very hard, standing under a warm shower, listening to very loud music, dancing to a CD or singing out loud.

If you have no planned distractions available, or if you are in a place where it is hard to do any of them, you can still practise paying mindful attention to whatever day-to-day activities you're doing: for example, focusing your entire attention on the physical sensations that accompany tasks such as walking to the shops, putting the washing out, doing the dishes, and so on. Again, the key thing is to pay mindful attention to the sensations or tasks.

**Mental distractions**

Paying mindful attention to your physical distractions can help shift your focus away from your distress. Your safe place imagery can also be used to provide a soothing distraction from painful thoughts and feelings. There is also a range of other mental distractions that people have found helpful.

Some of these are imagery exercises that focus on doing something with our distress to put it away from us – for example, imagining your painful emotions draining out of you like water out a pipe, or floating away like a balloon. Other people prefer the idea of putting their suffering away but knowing that they can come back to it at a later date – for example, imagining that it is in a box that they can lock away. Some like to leave their suffering with their compassionate companion.

Another technique is to practise bringing other thoughts to mind so that we give ourselves something else to focus on. These may be positive images of the future (for example, planning our next holiday) or of the past (for example, happy memories). Alternatively we can do impersonal mental tasks or puzzles, like a difficult chess or sudoko problem, or a mathematical task – even counting the bricks in a wall takes concentration and so can give temporary respite. Tasks which engage our imagination as well as our rational thoughts, such as following an absorbing book or TV programme, can also help to distract us.

## Emotional distractions

Often we find ourselves so caught up with our emotions that it is very difficult to find a way out of them, or indeed to feel that we have any control over our emotional state. At these times it can be helpful to break up these feelings in some way so that we can step outside them to explore compassionate ways to accept and manage them. Again, it can help to plan how you might do this before you get into an intense emotional state, and even to practise learning to switch your moods deliberately. This is very useful in giving you a greater sense of control over your feelings. You might want to start by getting into a positive mood, then interrupt it for a little while, and then bring it back again. A good way to do this is by using music or TV programmes. Start by listening to or watching something that makes you feel happy – perhaps an upbeat piece of music you really like, or a favourite comedy programme; them switch to something a little more sad – perhaps songs of unrequited love or a tearjerker; then play something that makes you happy again. Notice how your mood can change and how you can choose to allow yourself to go along with this.

You may wish to put together an 'emotional library' of music, films, books, soaps or art that you know can influence your mood. You can use this when you feel stuck with an emotion that you find distressing. It doesn't really matter what mood you use to switch out of this emotional state, as long as it is different from the one you are struggling with. For example, if you are feeling angry try not to watch a revenge film: you could watch something that frightens you, makes you cry or makes you laugh, so long as it doesn't exacerbate your feelings of anger, even on behalf of someone else!

The key to all of these distraction techniques is to find the ones that work for you, to have some available in advance, and to give yourself permission to use them as and when you need them. It can be really helpful to experiment with them when you don't need them. Avoid experimenting with them when you are feeling really upset. A good way to begin is to draw up a list of possibilities and try to practise a new one every day for a few days, until you find out which ones work best for you.

## Deciding to tolerate distress

Distress tolerance is a key element of compassion (take a look back at the 'compassion circle' in Figure 4.3). It is also a skill that most of us have to learn. When we are faced by difficult situations, setbacks or disappoint-ments, we are unlikely to think about how much distress we can tolerate: on the contrary, we are more likely to be thinking about how to *stop* feeling bad. So we will tend to rely on whatever way of doing this we've got used to – and if this is overeating, reaching for the chocolate bar or crisps, then so be it.

One of the things that a compassion focus can help us with is tolerating some degree of suffering in order to help us gain more control over whether to eat or not when the impulse arises. Now, of course, the key reason for learning to tolerate distress is to find new ways of coping with it, not simply to prove how much pain we can take! There will be some kinds of distress or discomfort that we can choose to subject ourselves to – as, for example, in giving up unhealthy eating habits; and there will be others – for example, resulting from an argument at work – that we may be able to plan for in advance. In both kinds of situation it can be helpful to use our compassion-ate mind to help us think about the pros and cons of tolerating the distress: for example, in the first case you might want to think about the possible benefits of tolerating the urge to reach for the chocolate bar without giving in to it. By acknowledging our desires in this way without responding to them, we can learn to act differently in the face of certain emotions.

Keep in mind that there can be many different emotions, at a range of different levels of intensity, that might be driving your eating. For example we can feel angry; fed up; deprived and deserving of food; lonely; or simply wanting to have a good time. And we can feel anything from mild irritation or frustration to utter misery or fury.

If you do decide to practise tolerating distress, be guided by the skills of self-compassion you learned earlier in this chapter. Don't set impossible goals, or see a return to your previous coping strategies as a failure. Your ability to tolerate distress is another 'mental ability' that you may need to develop slowly and to nurture. Here is an exercise that will help you to practise this useful skill.

## EXERCISE 6.1: LEARNING TO TOLERATE DISTRESS

Bring to mind your compassionate image – this can be either your compassionate self or your compassionate companion. Focus on a feeling of genuinely and kindly wanting to help yourself learn to understand the things that distress you, and to allow yourself to experience your emotions. What would your compassionate image say to help you allow yourself to face and explore your distress without resorting immediately to overeating or dieting?

You might want to include some of the things that people I have worked with have found helpful, for example:

- I am suffering these feelings for a reason, so in the future I will have these feelings less often.

- I am able to to experience my distress and to learn from it.

- My distress will pass; I can learn to ride out the wave.

- I am strong enough to bear my distress.

- This work is part of the long-term changes I can make to turn overeating into a thing of the past.

You can add anything else your compassionate image can think of in the space below:

- 

- 

- 

Thinking about the disadvantages of *not* tolerating your current distress can also be helpful. For example, you might call to mind what has happened in the past when you used overeating or dieting to escape the distress of the moment – perhaps feeling cross with yourself and even more distressed after overeating, or feeling first elated and then miserable after a diet that didn't last. However, if you do this, it is also important to remember that at that time you did not have the choices your new skills give you now – in other words, don't beat yourself up for having dealt with distress in the best way you could at the time.

So again, from the perspective of your compassionate image, try to write the downsides of not learning to tolerate your feelings in the space below:

- 

- 

- 

- 

- 

Next, try to make a plan for the type of feelings you want to learn to tolerate, and for how long. To start with you may want to work on the less painful or distressing feelings that you associate with overeating. For example, some people begin by working on tolerating the urge to overeat when they are happy or to reward themselves, and to aim at first to resist the urge to overeat for about five minutes. You may then decide to go ahead and eat, or you might decide to use some of the self-soothing or distraction activities that we explored earlier in this chapter. The point here is not to *stop* yourself overeating completely straight away, but to learn at least to *postpone* overeating for a fixed length of time. As you develop your confidence in your ability to tolerate and explore your feelings, you can work on tolerating more painful feelings and doing this for longer periods of time.

The key in this exercise is to use the time that you are tolerating these feelings to be mindful of the things that have caused you to overeat in the first place, perhaps even writing them down. Later in the book we will explore a more structured way of doing this by using a diary. On some days you will find tolerating your feelings easier than on others; as always, just go at your own pace and use your compassionate mind to guide you and help you to understand when and why the feelings you have arise.

# Compassionate thinking and behaviour

As we discovered in Chapter 4, the compassionate mind has a number of different elements, which we divided into 'attributes' and 'skills'. These relate both to our emotional and our rational minds, and to our actions: that is, to the way we feel, think and behave. So far we have been learning to bring our soothing system and compassionate emotions into play, using imagery to focus our compassionate attention on ourselves and others. In this section we will explore ways to develop our ability to think and act compassionately.

## Compassionate thinking

We have seen how the mindset we are in can affect the way we think about things. For example, if are in a dieting mindset we are more likely to think about the achievements that dieting will bring us, but also all the reasons why we think we need to lose weight, and to be very self-critical if we break our diet. If we are in a compassionate mindset, on the other hand, we are more likely to focus on our discomfort or distress and to look for ways to alleviate it with care and kindness. The aim of compassionate thinking is to help us stand back from the flow of our thoughts and think in a more balanced way, so that we are not too biased or at the mercy of our emotions.

### EXERCISE 6.2: COMPASSIONATE THOUGHT BALANCING

One way to develop our capacity for compassionate thinking is to note down the way we think when we are in different mindsets. We can then use our compassionate mind to develop other ways of thinking. Challenging our thinking can be very effective in helping us to learn to think differently. The key is not only to come up with alternative ways of thinking but also to express them compassionately. We can call this 'compassionate thought balancing'. You might like to give it a try now, using the examples set out in Figure 6.2. First imagine reading the 'compassionate alternative thoughts' out loud in a very critical or cold voice. Do you think someone would find this helpful? Now read the same thoughts out loud again, this time as if you really wanted to help and care for someone struggling with their overeating. Spend a few minutes thinking about the difference, and how you would feel about being on the receiving end of these things being said to you in the two different ways.

| Overeating thoughts | Compassionate alternative thoughts |
| --- | --- |
| There is something wrong with me because I overeat. | Overeating is very common. People overeat for a whole lot of reasons – because they are hungry, tired, upset or happy. Humans evolved to overeat, so it is normal to have the urge to. |
| I am weak because I overeat. | I don't want to overeat for lots of reasons, but stopping this is pretty tricky. It is a sign of how difficult my brain and body are to manage that I overeat, not a sign that I am weak. It takes a lot of strength and courage to want to work on giving up overeating. |
| I will never be able to stop overeating. | It is sad and frustrating that stopping overeating has been so difficult for me in the past. People can and do learn to change the way they eat and deal with their feelings but this will take some time. I can give myself the chance to see if the ways of doing it in the book can help me. |
| When I lose some weight I will start to make changes in my life and be happy. | Losing weight might happen if I stop overeating and dieting, but it is not fair to stop living my life until I lose some weight. I deserve to be happy and as healthy as I can be whatever my weight, and I am going to start doing things to care for myself regardless of my weight! |
| If I don't overeat I can't cope with my feelings. | It is OK to be worried about this; I have used overeating for years to help me manage my feelings. I can gradually learn to change this, but it is not the end of the world if I do need to overeat from time to time. I will get better at learning to manage my feelings the more I work on it. |
| I can't refuse to eat when everyone around me is eating. | Most people find this hard; after all eating is a very social thing. But I can choose when I eat – other people around me do choose not to eat at times and I don't think they are bad or rude. I can also choose to eat with them if I want, but perhaps eat a bit less than they do. |

**Figure 6.2:** Compassionate thought balancing: an example

Of course, learning to think and talk to yourself in this way, and then learning to believe your new thoughts, is a skill that you may need to practise. You can use the blank form in Worksheet 2 for this (there are a couple more blank sheets at the back of the book, and you can photocopy these if you need more). First write down your overeating (or dieting) thoughts in the left-hand column. You don't need to develop alternatives straight away. Sometimes we are so caught up in our usual mindsets that it is difficult to think differently. However, if you focus on your compassionate image or your compassionate self, using the exercises in Chapter 5, you will probably be able then to come back to your list and come up with alternative ways of thinking about these things. When you have finished, you can then practise reading them aloud. Choose the alternatives that you think are most likely to help you, and perhaps keep them with you, either written down on little 'flashcards' in your wallet or purse, or as texts to yourself, so you have them to hand to help you practise these new ways of thinking whenever thoughts that are likely to make you think about overeating crop up.

### EXERCISE 6.3: GETTING OUTSIDE YOUR MINDSET

Another way to develop your compassionate thinking is to explore the ways you normally think when you are in a particular mindset. For example, what kinds of thoughts do you have when you are in a 'dieting' mindset or a 'food as fun' mindset? You can start by jotting these down now. For example, in a dieting mindset you might think, 'I deserve to eat if I am unhappy,' 'Dieting will make me feel better about myself,' 'Overeating is something I can never resolve,' etc. Gently explore these thoughts, and see if you can develop compassionate alternatives by using your compassionate mind to try to answer the following questions.

- Is this thinking helpful to me?

- Would I think like this if I weren't in this (comfort eating/dieting/food as fun etc.) mindset?

- Would I teach a child or friend to think like this?

- If not, how would I like to teach them to think about these things?

**Worksheet 2: Compassionate thought balancing**

| Overeating thoughts | Compassionate alternative thoughts |
| --- | --- |
|  |  |

- How might I think about this when I am at my compassionate best?

- What would help me in the long run?

- Is this thinking compassionate?

The key point in this exercise is to try to be mindful of your thoughts and to see how they can be pulled in certain ways, depending on how you are feeling. This exercise will help you to stand back a little and observe your thoughts, enabling you to find a compassionate, fair and balanced approach.

## Self-critical thinking versus self-compassionate self-correction

Some people believe that self-criticism is the only way to make themselves do things, succeed or be good. For example, a person might say, 'If I didn't kick myself, I'd never stop eating.' Or they might believe that unless they are critical and 'keep themselves on their toes', they will be lazy, and so they use self-bullying and self-criticism to drive themselves on. Some people learn self-criticism in childhood, if they have had parents and teachers who tended to focus more on their errors than on the things they did well and the good things about them. As a result, the child becomes good at self-criticism and self-punishment, but poor at seeing their own good points and not used to rewarding and valuing themselves. However, it's not always the case that self-criticism is learned in childhood: it is important to remember that criticism based on shaming is very common in our society. We are likely to experience it at school, but we can also see it in our treatment of the mistakes of politicians and celebrities in our daily papers. So even if we don't have direct experience of frequent criticism as we're growing up, there is so much of it around us that it can be hard for us to develop other ways of relating to ourselves.

Of course, there will be times when things we do don't go as we would like them to, and when we want to change what we do for the better. Compassion is certainly not about an 'anything goes' approach! So what we are aiming at is a way of correcting ourselves kindly and gently, with compassion, and understanding that change is often a difficult and long-term process.

| Compassionate self-correction is focused on: | Shame-based self-criticism is focused on: |
|---|---|
| • the desire to improve<br>• growth and enhancement<br>• looking forward<br>• encouragement, support and kindness<br>• building on positives (e.g. seeing what one did well and then considering learning points)<br>• focusing on specific areas and qualities of self<br>• focusing on and hoping for success<br>• increasing the chances of engagement | • the desire to condemn and punish<br>• punishing past errors and often looking backwards<br>• anger, frustration, contempt and disappointment<br>• focusing on faults and fear of being found out<br>• focusing on the whole self<br>• focusing on fear of failure<br>• increasing chances of avoidance and withdrawal |

**Figure 6.3:** Compassionate self-correction versus shame-based self-criticism

*Source*: Adapted with permission from P. Gilbert, *The Compassionate Mind* (London: Constable & Robinson, 2009).

It can be helpful to keep the differences between shame-based self-criticism or self-attacking and compassion-based self-correction to hand so that you can more easily work out which one you're using when you try to correct yourself. The key differences are summarized in Figure 6.3.

You can see that shame-based self-criticism involves the emotions associated with the threat system, such as anger and fear. Letting go of this type of self-criticism can help you to learn new ways to manage your feelings and to deal with the urges and desires that cause you to overeat. Compassionate self-correction focuses on and encourages your real desire to do your best and to improve.

To see how this works, consider two sports coaches teaching a young child. One focuses on their faults and picks on them when they make mistakes. The other focuses on what the child does well, encourages the child to improve and learn from their mistakes, and offers clear guidance. Which one will help the child's confidence? Which one is the child more likely to want to work? Which one do you prefer? Attacking self-criticism can often make us feel disheartened so that we just want to give up and hide away. If we really want to reduce our overeating (or correct other aspects of our behaviour), we stand a better chance of doing so if we get into the habit of using *compassionate* self-correction when things go wrong or when we start to feel frustrated with ourselves.

Compassionate self-correction is based on being mindful, open-hearted and honest about our mistakes, acknowledging our genuine wish to learn from them. No one wakes up in the morning and thinks to themselves, 'Oh, I think I will make a real cock-up of my eating today, just for the hell of it.' Most of us would like eat healthily, most of us would like to avoid mistakes, most of us would like to avoid being out of control with our temper and so on. Compassionate self-correction recognizes this. Self-criticism, on the other hand, deals in fear and anger: it is concerned with punishment for things we have already done. The problem is that we cannot change a single moment of the past; we can only change the future, and beating ourselves up is really not the best way of helping ourselves to do better.

Making the transition from shame-based self-criticism to compassion-based self-correction can be difficult at first, but with practice it will become easier. You may well already be turning more readily to compassionate thoughts as a result of your imagery work, and it can be really helpful to keep a note of them as they develop, perhaps even keeping the list with you to look at when you are tempted to return to self-criticism. Later on we will look at how we can develop this supportive practice of compassionate self-correction using techniques such as compassionate letter-writing, which is described in detail in Chapter 14.

## Compassionate behaviour

Behaving compassionately is doing helpful, kind or thoughtful things to help ourselves and others to deal with difficulties, setbacks and suffering, and to develop, flourish and improve.

Many people with eating problems have told me that they have been able to *act* in more compassionate ways before they can routinely *think* in a compassionate way. This takes us back to the comparison with 'method acting' I suggested when introducing the imagery work in Chapter 5: it's often the case that *doing* things compassionately for ourselves will not necessarily be associated with the *feelings* of self-compassion, at least in the early stages. As I've said before, this is just fine: it is our intentions and our behaviours that matter; the feelings can and will come along later.

Learning to behave compassionately towards yourself can help maintain your compassionate motivation. There will, of course, be times when you're angry or frustrated and don't want to carry through on your commitment to looking after yourself properly. This is entirely understandable; but if you can, to the best of your ability, just notice and be compassionate to your anger and frustration, and act compassionately towards yourself – it will be easier to pick yourself up and carry on. Sometimes we just need to ride out the waves of emotion and wait for the intensity of our feelings to subside.

In later chapters of this book we will be working on developing compassionate behaviour in relation to your eating and your body's needs for activity and rest. For now, you might want to try practising acting compassionately towards yourself for perhaps five minutes every day. If you are one of the many people who find it harder to be kind to themselves than to others, you might find it easier to approach this by doing something compassionate for another person or animal for the first week and then gradually adding things you do for yourself after this.

Before you actually try to do this, it can be helpful to put together a list of things that you have done, or seen others do, that you consider to be compassionate. You might also find it helpful to talk to people you know, or to notice what they do, to find out how they are kind to themselves. Below are some ideas to get you started:

- Do one thing, no matter how small, which is specifically designed to be enjoyable (for example, take a warm, scented bath).

- Make time to speak kindly to someone. Try to find out a little bit about them.

- Each day do one spontaneous act of kindness for someone else that doesn't involve food or eating.

- Practise one act of forgiveness to yourself, no matter how small, especially if you tried something and weren't as successful as you wanted to be, or if you had a relapse of some kind.

- Set time aside to practise some of your self-compassion or distress management exercises.

- Spend five minutes remembering kindnesses that occurred in the day.

## Keeping diaries of your practice

People often keep diaries to record their thoughts and feelings, especially if they're feeling low. Keeping a diary of all your practice with compassion can be really helpful in enabling you to see how you are getting on. You can use it to record the specific exercises you do from this book, but also to keep notes of your occasional practice, your personal observations, what your compassionate mind says, and your successes, no matter how small. This can help you to keep track of your progress and to see which of the exercises are turning out to be most helpful for you. Figure 6.4 shows an example of a week's completed practice diary, and Worksheet 3 gives you a blank form that you can use for your own diary if you wish. (There are a couple more copies at the back of the book.)

## Blocks to compassion

Remember David, whom we met in Chapter 3? He had lost a lot of weight after a period of illness, and then had got stuck in a cycle of yo-yo dieting and self-recrimination. His reactions when he began to work on self-compassion were typical of many. David recognized that dieting had made him feel better about himself, helping him feel in control and more confident. Looking back at the past, he came to see how his eating habits had changed alongside the events in his life, and this helped him to realize how he had come to rely on overeating to manage some very difficult experiences in his past. However, although he could see the logic of why overeating had helped him, he could not stop criticizing himself for his 'weakness' in needing food to comfort him, or for the unintended conse-quences of overeating, such as weight gain. David also found it very

**Worksheet 3: My compassion practice diary**

| Day | Type of practice, time and how long for | Comments: what was helpful? |
|---|---|---|
| Monday | | |
| Tuesday | | |
| Wednesday | | |
| Thursday | | |
| Friday | | |
| Saturday | | |
| Sunday | | |
| Comments on week's practice | | |

*Source:* Reproduced with kind permission from the Compassionate Mind Foundation website.

| Day | Type of practice, time and for how long | Comments: what was helpful? |
|---|---|---|
| Thursday | 10 a.m.<br>Soothing breathing rhythm<br>Compassionate self | Felt calmer, less stressed. Noticed mind wandering but managed to keep focusing on breathing.<br>Tricky to get started but began to see the point – thought about someone I wanted to be compassionate to. |
| Friday | Soothing breathing in bed<br>Compassionate self on the bus | Mixed today as busy.<br>Useful to slow down and refocus and think about the self I would like to be. Able to get in touch with a desire in myself to be kind and calm. Recognized that I can be quite self-critical, but can slow down and refocus. |
| Saturday | Very busy<br>In the bath – 15 mins<br>compassionate relaxing | Did occasionally think about being mindful and taking a moment to 'slow down'. Also thought about my compassionate colour . . . But lots to do with the family.<br>Only thought about it towards the end. |
| Sunday | Very busy with family so no specific time | Trying to think about compassion at different points in the day. |
| Monday | 11 a.m. – half hour focused on both compassionate self and compassionate imagery | Recognize I need to spend time to practise. When I can make time it does help.<br>Working with my image was difficult, it tended to come and go, but just allowed that to happen and began to have a sense of an image rather than seeing anything clearly. |

| Tuesday | Similar to Monday |
| --- | --- |
| Wednesday | 2 p.m. – compassionate self | Have a friend who's been having difficulties so practised imagining compassionate self and just being compassionate to her. Felt I could sense this desire in me for her to feel better. Recognizing I do have compassionate feelings. |
| Comments on week's practice | Trying to bring my practice into every day life as well as setting time aside. Recognizing that it's about remembering to attend and focus on compassionate things. |

**Figure 6.4:** Compassion practice diary: an example

*Source:* Reproduced with kind permission from the Compassionate Mind Foundation website.

difficult to be compassionate with himself over the difficult events in his life. He could see that if they had happened to someone else he would feel sad for them and angry on their behalf and would want to help them, but he felt nothing for himself. When I expressed my compassion for the difficult experiences he had had, David found this very difficult to accept – he even talked about ending our work together, as he felt he did not deserve and could not cope with other people caring for him.

Fortunately, David was able to explore and overcome some his blocks to compassion using the exercises set out in this section of the chapter. At first he was not able to *feel* compassion for himself, but he was prepared to have a go at *behaving* compassionately. He found that this helped him to recognize the positive changes in his mood and eating that caring for himself gave him, and he gradually learned to value his capacity for self-compassion.

Just like David, many of us are not used to thinking compassionately about ourselves, and some of us find it difficult to accept and use compassion offered by others. There can be many reasons for this. Some of them are the result of the culture that we live in; others may be related to painful experiences in our past or present. In this section we will explore some of the most common blocks to allowing ourselves to accept compassion from others, and to offering it to ourselves.

These common blocks to compassion include:

- confusing compassion with pity;

- feeling that those who need compassion are weak;

- seeing acceptance of compassion as self-indulgent or selfish;

- seeing compassion as a soft option;

- seeing compassion as letting one's guard down or letting oneself off the hook;

- believing that compassion means getting rid of feelings (for example, never feeling angry if people upset or hurt you).

For some people, the idea of compassion can trigger difficult emotionally charged memories or strong feelings that can also act as blocks. These include:

- anger for a lack of compassion experienced either now or in the past;

- grief for pain they have been through or are going through now;

- fear or anxiety – either that compassion will be taken away, or that it will come at a cost.

Many people find one or more of these blocks getting in the way of their work on developing self-compassion skills and accepting compassion from others, even others they know they can trust. Of course, some people may simply never have thought that they might be able to use this aspect of their personality to help themselves as well as other people, possibly because they have found other coping strategies (like comfort eating or dieting) to be effective. If this is the case for you, or if you don't have any blocks to compassion, you may wish to skip the exercises in the rest of this chapter and move straight on to the next chapter. However, if you have any concerns about developing your compassionate mind, for any reason, it might be a good idea to try these four exercises before you move on. Also, if you find that blocks come up when you try any of the other exercises in the book, you can come back to these exercises to help you work through them.

Before using the exercises to explore your own blocks to self-compassion, it may be helpful to consider some of the common blocks in a little more detail.

## Confusing compassion with pity

Although compassion can bring to the fore our sympathy and desire to alleviate distress, unlike pity it also recognizes our own and other people's wisdom, courage and resilience. Compassion starts from a recognition that in our common humanity we can all, at times, struggle to cope with life. Pitying other people, by contrast, tends be associated with feeling superior to them. Thus many people have a strong aversion to being pitied, associating it with being seen as inferior or weak. Compassion combines sympathy with respect.

## Feeling that those who need compassion are weak

Interestingly, we tend not to think in this way when we offer compassion to others. We see them as in a temporary state of suffering, which we may be able to help relieve. We are more likely to think that *we* are weak if we need compassion. This may be related to the emphasis our modern culture places on self-sufficiency, or to concerns about what other people will do if we show them any sign of 'weakness'. This is often related to the confusion of compassion with pity, noted above.

## Seeing acceptance of compassion as self-indulgent or selfish

When we are compassionate towards others, we tend to put their needs first. Thus many of us recoil from the idea that self-compassion may involve putting our own needs first, having been brought up to believe that this is wrong. In fact, however, allowing ourselves to experience compassion from others, or giving it to ourselves, is often an important step in enabling us to be *more* concerned for others. For example, when we are in stuck in a comfort food mindset we can be very single-minded about eating, and when we are stuck in a dieting mindset we may think about little other than our diet. In both cases, this narrow focus may mean that we unintentionally neglect the needs of others because we are just not aware of them. Opening ourselves to compassion, as we have seen, can also mean that we will be more open to being compassionate with others.

## Seeing compassion as a soft option

Actually, developing self-compassion is hard work! Self-compassion requires us to develop the courage to address our difficulties, which often involves facing problems that we have used our dieting or comfort eating mindsets to avoid because we felt we could not cope with them. It also encourages us to face up to and take responsibility for our actions, including those that hurt ourselves or others. Self-compassion can also require us to be assertive with others, for example resisting the urge to eat if they offer us food that we don't want to eat.

Before you begin the next group of four exercises you may want to start with a brief period of reflection – just a minute or so – on a time when you experienced compassion from others, or tried to offer yourself compassion, as in Exercises 5.9 and 5.12 in the previous chapter. Notice the thoughts and feelings that come up as you do this and try to jot them down. After about a minute, use your soothing breathing rhythm to help refocus your attention and step out of the reflection.

The four exercises are presented here as a group, but you may want to do each one separately, and to plan in something soothing or distracting to do after you finish each exercise.

### EXERCISE 6.4: MY PERSONAL BLOCKS TO EXPERIENCING COMPASSION FROM OTHERS

Please list here any thoughts or ideas that you think might stop you letting other people offer you compassion. You might find it helpful to take a look back at the common blocks listed at the beginning of this section.

- 
- 
- 
- 
- 

### EXERCISE 6.5: MY PERSONAL BLOCKS TO DEVELOPING SELF-COMPASSION

Please list here any thoughts or ideas that you think might prevent you being compassionate towards yourself. Again, you might find it helpful to take a look back at the common blocks listed at the beginning of this section.

- 
- 
- 
- 
- 

When you have done both these exercises, it can be helpful to consider the blocks you have identified from the perspective of your compassionate image. What might they suggest as reasons why you have these blocks? You might even try writing a compassionate letter about your blocks to allowing yourself to experience compassion. (For detailed guidance on how to go about this, see Chapter 14.) Your letter may help you to find ways around these blocks.

If you wish, you can use the next two exercises to draw together your thoughts on how you might manage these blocks. Again, you can use your compassionate image to help you.

### EXERCISE 6.6: COPING WITH BLOCKS TO COMPASSION FROM OTHERS

Please try to list anything you could do or say to help you cope with your blocks to accepting compassion from others.

- 
- 
- 
- 
- 

### EXERCISE 6.7: COPING WITH BLOCKS TO SELF-COMPASSION

Please try to list anything you could do or say to help you cope with your blocks to accepting compassion from yourself.

- 
- 
- 
- 
- 

Another way around these blocks is simply to note these beliefs as common, but to practise compassion anyway. Think of it like physiotherapy. If you had a weak muscle in your leg, perhaps as a result of injury, you wouldn't tell yourself that you didn't deserve to have a stronger muscle. So why not build up your compassionate skills anyway, and then, if you decide you don't want to use them, that's up to you. However, you can only *choose* not to be self-compassionate if you have the ability to be self-compassionate, and so to make that genuine choice you will need to learn the skills.

Earlier in this chapter we explored learning how to tolerate distress. If you are not used to receiving compassion, or have a lot of blocks to this, you may also find that this skill can also help you to 'get used to' compassion. Perhaps you can work out how much compassion you can let yourself have by using Exercise 5.9 from the previous chapter, or deciding to tolerate other people's kindness to you.

---

### SUMMARY

In this chapter we have explored some additional ways of managing feelings of discomfort and distress. It can be useful to keep a record of those that you find most helpful and the situations in which they're most likely to be effective. This way you can build up a toolkit of new ways of coping with the situations and experiences that trouble you before we begin work on changing your eating habits.

Many of us find it difficult to allow ourselves to experience compassion from other people and – particularly – from ourselves, and we have also explored this difficulty a little further in this chapter. It's important to remember that it's very common to experience blocks to compassion, but that we can learn to think and behave in more compassionate ways even before we learn to feel compassion, and so can make progress in developing these key skills that will help us to deal with the problem of overeating.

# 7 Why do we overeat?
A compassionate mind approach

Before you start working on a more compassionate mind approach to your eating and your body, it can be very helpful to understand why you overeat now. The particular reasons that apply in your individual case may include events and influences in the past, as well as factors present in the here and now. This chapter guides you through a way of identifying these influences and making sense of them. In the next chapter we will focus more on how things in your past may have made you vulnerable to overeating; then, in Chapter 9, we will look more closely at the 'here-and-now' factors before moving on to consider how you can put all this information together into a personal formulation that will be the basis of your work to beat your overeating for good.

This chapter is a little different from the previous ones in that it involves you doing quite a lot of thinking and reflecting on how and why you eat. This can be an emotional journey for some people. Coming to an understanding of how and why we sometimes eat too much can involve remembering difficult experiences with food and our bodies in the past, and perhaps grieving for the pain and distress we have unintentionally put ourselves through in trying to follow eating regimes that were – though we didn't know it at the time – inevitably doomed to failure. You may also find that you have used food to punish or reward yourself for things that have happened in your life. It's because these explorations are likely to bring up quite a lot of emotion that it's really helpful to approach them with compassion – and this is where you'll see all the work you have already done paying off in helping you through the next stages.

So, with each of the exercises in this chapter, only go at a pace you can manage. Kindly and gently accept your emotional reactions: if you're upset, confused or angry, or even proud of the short bursts of control you have had over your eating using diets in the past, that's fine. But remember: although there will come a time for compassionate self-correction, there is no place in the compassionate mind approach for shaming self-criticism. Beating yourself up for the way you have felt, or for the ways you have tried to manage your feelings in the past, *will not help* and can make you feel worse. Compassionately acknowledge that you are showing strength and courage now in trying to find new ways of dealing with the challenges of life, including managing our 'see-food-and-eat-it' brain in a world of plenty.

So this may be a difficult journey – but the rewards can be amazing. Many people say that this process of self-discovery has been crucial in helping them to understand their relationship with food and eating, and from there to take responsibility for changing that relationship.

There are six golden rules for undertaking this journey:

- Make practical and emotional space for doing each exercise.

- Expect the exercises to be challenging but not overwhelming.

- Be as honest with yourself as you can.

- Use other people to help and support you if they are available and interested – this can include family, friends or medical professionals.

- Expect it to take time to use your new knowledge to change the way you act.

- Remember that understanding things now does not mean you could have changed the way you behaved in the past, or altered the events that happened to you.

You might find it helpful to write these down in your notebook, or take a copy of them, and just remind yourself of them each time you move on to tackle a new exercise.

## What a compassionate 'formulation' for overeating involves

In approaching overeating with compassion, we are trying to understand the factors that have influenced who we have become and why we act as we do. We know, for example, that if you grow up in a particular (say) religious group it's likely that you will adopt values and attitudes shared by that group. If you grow up in a loving environment it's likely that you'll feel confident about yourself; whereas if you grow up in a hostile or neglectful environment or are bullied at school, you're likely to feel less confident about yourself and more fearful or suspicious of others around you.

Now, of course, not all our difficulties are related to our childhoods – many relate quite simply to where we are now – but childhood is important and can create in us certain assumptions and values, ways of behaving and ways of dealing with emotions such as fear, loneliness, anxiety and anger – and these can have their effects on our attitudes and values to do with eating.

The compassionate mind approach to therapy considers how the emotional and psychological problems we have now may have developed through a series of experiences and reactions over time. In this approach we begin by thinking about some of the key childhood experiences that might have had an influence on our sense of self and the things we are sensitive to. Anything that we felt as threatening can be especially significant – for example, criticism from or rejection by others. Also, anything that aroused feelings of shame – a sense that we are inferior, inadequate or no good in some way – is also significant, because once we have learned to feel ashamed we can carry this feeling, or a fear of its returning, around with us for a long time. And the shame, or the fear of it, can very easily can come to the surface when we make mistakes, get criticized – or lose control of our eating.

So our compassionate mind approach will first try to establish what our underlying feelings about ourselves are, and where they might have come from. The next part of the exploration concerns the *safety strategies* we have developed to defend ourselves against these unpleasant feelings – for example, of threat, fear or shame. These are ways in which our minds will try to avoid experiencing these uncomfortable emotions, or coping with them if we can't prevent them. So, for example, somebody who was bullied at school and felt ashamed of her body weight might learn to become quite submissive in order not to make others angry. She might also become preoccupied with her appearance. If someone feels overwhelmed by painful emotions, he might try to avoid them by turning to food (or other substances such as alcohol) to calm and distract himself. If these safety strategies work, even if only in the short term, people will tend to use them over and over again. This is, of course, very understandable, but it prevents them from addressing the original difficulty – and also tends, as we saw in Chapter 6, to reinforce the mistaken belief that those painful emotions should not, indeed cannot, be tolerated.

In addition to identifying safety strategies, a compassionate formulation of the reasons for overeating will investigate the ways in which we try to correct our mistakes, avoid problems or deal with frustration. It is sadly very common for people to become very self-critical when things go wrong for them, particularly if they can't work out why this is happening. For example, we may often criticize ourselves because we're disappointed that we can't *make ourselves* do better. This self-criticism can be partly linked to fear of the consequences of not dealing with the problem. It can also be linked to memories of people being critical and cruel in the past. Sometimes one's own critical voice sounds remarkably like that of a parent or teacher or school bully. We often think that self-criticism is somehow going to improve ourselves – but in fact it's more likely just to make us feel more ashamed.

## Eating as a safety strategy

We create safety strategies to deal with things in our internal world – things that go on in our own heads, such as avoiding difficult emotions or trying to stimulate pleasurable emotions – and of course things that go on in the outside world, such as trying to avoid rejection or getting people to like us and be kind to us. The trouble is that the safety strategies we come up with as solutions can also become part of the problem. For example, imagine the difficulties somebody who's always submissive is going to run into, or those that will confront somebody who never wants to confront an uncomfortable emotion. So safety strategies can have *unintended consequences*.

Now, as we have already seen, we may overeat or diet, and find our weight going up and down like a yo-yo, for a variety of reasons. This may happen, for example:

- because we don't know enough about the way our eating patterns affect our weight;

- because of how the things that we consume other than food affect our appetite and our ability to regulate it;

- because of habits we learned while we were growing up.

However, overeating can also be a *safety strategy*, which can serve a very useful purpose in helping us to regulate our emotions, and particularly in helping us to manage the things that bother us most – our 'key threats', if you like. When overeating has become a way of dealing with our emotions it's important to recognize this, because if we're going to have a good chance of succeeding in changing our eating habits we're going to need to work on the issues that drive it. For example, if we have an underlying sense of shame or of being out of control, simply trying to change our eating behaviour without changing those feelings may by tricky. Indeed, when we begin to challenge and work on our safety strategies, some of the key threats they were designed to deal with can resurface – so we're going to have to deal with them!

As the term implies, *safety strategies* are designed to keep us safe in some way. They can be deliberate and thought-out, or they can also be things that we find ourselves doing without really knowing why. They fall into two categories: *external safety strategies*, which are aimed at managing how other people will see us or treat us; and *internal safety strategies*, which are about managing our own emotions and how we think or feel about ourselves.

Figure 7.1 shows you how safety strategies are developed in response to 'key threats', both past and present; how they have both intended and unintended consequences; and how these consequences keep the safety strategies in use. We can call the overall pattern a 'compassionate formulation for overeating'. To give you a better idea of how this works in

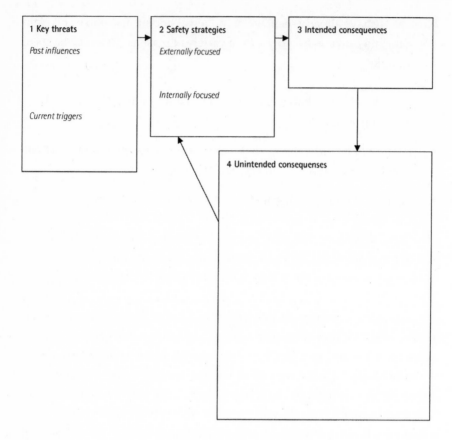

**Figure 7.1:** A compassionate formulation for overeating

practice, we're now going to look at Alison's 'compassionate formulation for overeating', which is summarized in Figure 7.2.

# Exploring Alison's compassionate formulation for overeating

## Key threats: past influences

Alison recalled that when she was growing up her parents were very loving, but set quite high standards for her. They appeared disappointed if she failed at things and at times were difficult to please. They were busy

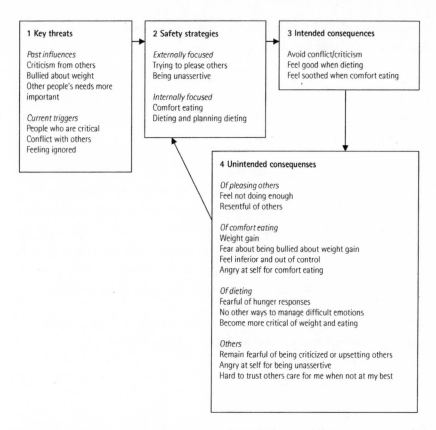

**Figure 7.2:** Alison's compassionate formulation for overeating

people and she had to work hard to earn their attention. She remembered dreading any criticism intruding on the precious moments of loving attention she had from them. She doesn't recall much open or affectionate discussion of her feelings in any depth, learning that in life you 'just get on with things'. She also remembered that she had to work quite hard to succeed at things, as she was not a naturally gifted student. Alison recalled that her parents would be proud of her when she achieved things, but she was always worried that they would criticize her if she failed.

So Alison developed a belief that people liked and cared about you if you weren't a nuisance to them and just got on with things and achieved things. She was very anxious about what other people thought about her when she wasn't able to do this. In her heart she felt that other people saw her as a disappointment, and would want to distance themselves from her rather than help if she failed or made mistakes.

Sadly, the belief that love, approval or support will only be offered to us if we 'deserve' them is very common – a lot more common than most of us imagine. Many of us worry that if we struggle or fall over very few genuine helping hands will come to our aid.

We can think about the beliefs Alison developed in terms of the three systems of emotional regulation that we discussed in Chapter 3. (You might want to look back at Figure 3.1 on page 54.) Alison's sense of security has come to be based upon her ability to maintain her drive and achievement system. Only then does she begin to feel safe and less fearful of others. She doesn't find it easy to get access to her soothing system (through being kind to herself or expecting others to be kind to her).

Alison also remembered being slightly overweight as a child and being bullied for several years when she moved to secondary school. She felt herself to be a very caring person and felt that other people's needs should take priority over her own.

## Key threats: current triggers

By exploring her personal history in this way, Alison came to recognize that as an adult she found it very difficult to deal with being criticized, or with situations where she might be criticized. She found conflict with others very difficult and struggled to be assertive about her needs. She also noticed that feeling that other people had overlooked or ignored her left her feeling angry towards them.

Alison began to recognize that one of the reasons why she didn't like any kind of conflict and could easily feel overwhelmed by it was that she had different feelings going on at the same time. For example, she was clearly anxious about the rejection of being put down, but there was also an element of anger in the background because she wanted to defend herself – and yet she was also anxious about this anger in case other people would see her as silly. So she also tended to criticize herself for feeling angry. So you won't be surprised to hear that anger was a feeling Alison struggled with and tried to avoid. And you can probably guess what she did if she got angry – she ate.

## Safety strategies

Alison saw that she had tried to avoid conflict and criticism mainly by trying to predict the needs of others, especially those in authority or who had some power over her, and to please them. Typically, she found that if the emotional temperature in a potential conflict was rising she would immediately get anxious and back off, falling into a submissive attitude. That safety strategy was so well rehearsed that it was automatic for her, and even though she found herself battling with it at times she was also frightened to overrule it. She also recognized how both comfort eating and dieting had helped her to manage the threat of criticism.

So Alison noticed that she had three main safety strategies, which she called 'pleasing others', 'comfort eating' and 'dieting'. Pleasing others is an example of an external safety strategy. Comfort eating was an internal safety strategy, designed to help Alison cope with or turn off painful feelings. Dieting was both an external safety strategy (helping her to manage her fear of criticism from others) and an internal safety strategy (helping to improve her feelings about herself and to give her a sense of achievement).

## Intended consequences

The consequences Alison intended to follow from dieting were feeling better about herself and avoiding distressing thoughts about feeling inferior, out of control, criticized or in conflict with others. Comfort eating had the intended consequences of helping her to deal with distressing emotions (particularly anger) when these thoughts did arise by soothing her. Being unassertive helped her to avoid conflict with and criticism from others.

## Unintended consequences

Let's look at the unintended consequences of Alison's safety strategies in more detail. It is common for these consequences, which we don't plan or foresee, to maintain or even worsen the difficulties we have.

### Pleasing others

Alison found that pleasing others covered a numbers of things she did to avoid being criticized. These included overworking, trying to predict and meet the needs of others, always putting her needs second, being unassertive and avoiding conflict. The unintended consequences of these strategies were that she felt hurried and put upon, never achieving quite enough, somehow a failure and inadequate, yet also resentful of the demands that others put on her and the effects that meeting their needs had on her physical, emotional and social life.

### Comfort eating

Alison noticed that comfort eating really helped her to soothe her distress (an intended consequence). Looking back, she noticed that this pattern had begun relatively early in life and may have contributed to her being slightly overweight between the ages of ten and sixteen (an unintended consequence). She worried that gaining weight through comfort eating would lead to her be bullied again, and these worries often brought back the memories, and associated distress, of the times when she had been bullied about her weight in the past. As her weight increased so her mood would dip. The self-critical voice within her would start up again and she would be angry with herself for being unable to control her urges to eat.

### Dieting

Alison remembered that dieting was initially a way to help her to lose some weight to avoid being bullied and to give her a feeling of being in control and to some degree a sense of pride and pleasure in her appearance. Her plans to diet would be triggered by becoming more aware than usual of her weight and shape (noticing, for example, that her jeans and dresses were getting tight), and more critical of her appearance. However, she also found it difficult to cope with feeling hungry, and would get angry with herself when she was tempted to break her diet.

When Alison was dieting she could not turn to comfort eating to cope with difficult emotions in her life. This meant that her feelings of anger and irritation with herself (either because of her weight or at being hungry) were with her even more. Alison found that planning a diet could give her hope about managing her weight, and distracted her from these feelings temporarily. But then thoughts about dieting tended to intrude at other times in her life. For example, her mind often wandered to thoughts about losing weight when she was trying to concentrate on tasks at work, and often she would find herself seeking reassurance from her partner that her diet was working – which he found quite irritating!

## All safety strategies

Alison recognized that together, her safety strategies had the unintended consequence of not allowing her to develop other ways to manage her fear of being criticized, her inability to assert herself and her anger and irritation towards others. She also noticed that she was often angry or disappointed with herself for needing to comfort eat, diet, or avoid conflict and criticism and that this tended to lower her mood, even when she had supportive friends or family around her. These unintended consequences left Alison feeling even more distressed and needing her safety strategies even more to help her to cope with her emotions.

Working out this 'formulation' of threats, safety strategies and intended and unintended consequences helped Alison to understand where her tendency to overeat had come from, but also, and more importantly, it helped her to make sense of why it had been so difficult to give it up over the years, even though she really wanted to.

Having got to this point, Alison could begin to offer herself compassion for the pain she had experienced in the past and to recognize that overeating had been the best way she could help herself cope with that pain and to function in the world. Having compassionately acknowledged this, she could go on to explore new ways to address her key fears without using her old safety strategies and so work towards breaking out of the vicious circle of overeating.

## Why draw up a compassionate formulation for overeating?

It's important to think through why we want to set out a formulation like this, and how it relates to the compassionate mind approach we've discussed in earlier chapters of this book. We begin with a genuine desire to develop wisdom and insight into our difficulties. The process of building our formulation allows us to stand back and see how different pieces of our lives fit together. When we began to put together Alison's formulation, she could see how the difficulties she got into arose from the combination of her experiences in life. By the time the formulation was complete we could also see that Alison was likely to become even more stuck in her current vicious circle if she went on criticizing and blaming herself for her difficulties and how she copes with them.

To sum up, then, setting out a compassionate formulation for our overeating has a number of benefits:

- It allows us to be open and honest without blaming ourselves.

- It can help us to recognize that our overeating is the result of many complex and interacting factors.

- It can help us to see more clearly how our overeating works, including all the intended and unintended consequences of overeating.

- It can help us recognize that although it is not our fault that we overeat (because we are 'set up' for it in so many ways), it *is* our responsibility to resolve it.

- It can help us to think carefully, from a kind, encouraging and supportive perspective, about how to move forward to being the kind of person we want to be and coping with things in our lives in a way that we're happy with.

- It can help us to acknowledge the need for compassion, understanding and encouragement on our journey towards becoming that person.

- It can help us to think about and plan which aspects of our overeating to work on first.

- It can help us to see if the work we are doing is successfully tackling the factors that trigger our overeating and keep it going.

Always keep in mind that this is a *compassionate* formulation, developed from within a compassionate mindset; that is, from a genuine intention and desire to understand and care for ourselves. It is not another tool with which to beat ourselves up for failure or non-achievement!

## Making your own compassionate formulation

A compassionate formulation is always a 'best guess' at how our difficulties have evolved and what keeps us stuck. In the coming chapters we will explore in more detail different ways to make sense of the past and present influences on your overeating. For now we are going to work though the process of constructing a compassionate formulation for your overeating using things you already know about yourself. So we are going to spend a little time thinking about how some of the things that trigger your overeating or shift you into dieting are related to underlying fears and worries that you might be carrying over from the past.

Bear in mind that these are just ideas to help you think through your own formulation. Keep in mind, too, that this is a *compassionate* approach, so you will be thinking about this in a compassionate, friendly way, curious and open to discovery, rather than judging and critical, recognizing that all human beings struggle with a combination of the same range of emotions and their own individual life histories. See your discoveries as ways of understanding yourself better and also perhaps working, step by step, towards making decisions about how you would like to change things – how you would like to become kinder and more forgiving to yourself and at the same time more encouraging, more supportive of change and growth – giving yourself that kind arm around your shoulder.

There are three exercises below that you might wish to try to help you develop your own formulation. Take a little while to read them through first. And take your time working through them – there is no rush. This framework will be the basis for much of the work you will do on changing your eating, so you deserve the time and space to put it together thoughtfully and, if this is more comfortable for you, bit by bit. So do the exercises below at a pace you can manage.

Before you attempt any of the exercises, be sure to bring your compassionate image alongside you. If you find while you are doing an exercise that you are becoming self-critical or that the exercise is too much for you to manage, step way from the exercise and bring your compassionate mind back to the fore before going any further. Just to remind you, the best way to do this is to begin by establishing your soothing breathing rhythm or safe place image. When you feel ready you can then bring up your compassionate image (either 'you at your best' or your compassionate companion). When you have the image in mind, spend a little time exploring what it feels like to step into the shoes and role of your compassionate image; what it feels like to be strong, warm, caring, interested in developing and fostering the potential of another human being. Notice how this changes your emotions, the things you would pay attention to and the ways you would think and act. When you have a sense of this you can then imagine what answers they would give to the questions in the exercises as they try to help you develop a personal formulation for your difficulties.

### EXERCISE 7.1: TALKING TO YOUR COMPASSIONATE IMAGE

Imagine that you're talking to your compassionate image or your very best friend and explaining to them some of the things in your early life that you think might have set you up for the difficulties with eating you have now. Remember, if this becomes overwhelming or too upsetting for you then it's quite OK to back off for a while and come back to it when you are ready. The idea of the task is not to distress you, but to give you a compassionate lens through which you can look at possible connections between your past and your present. This is why imagining you're talking to a deeply compassionate person can be very helpful.

### EXERCISE 7.2: WRITING A COMPASSIONATE LIFE STORY

It is sometimes helpful to write a compassionate life story – as if you were writing a letter about yourself to someone. If you want to try this, you might find it helpful to have some questions in your mind to get you started. These can include:

- What were the most important influences on me while I was growing up?

- What are the key distressing emotional memories that may have affected me? These are memories of important events or relationships in your life; they often come to mind when we are threatened, and may be linked to our drive/achievement system or trigger difficult feelings in us (such as shame or anger).

- What threats, worries and uncertainties about myself carry through into today from my early life?

- How have I learned to cope with things that frighten me? If I had to guess, what might my basic safety strategies be?

- When confronted with setbacks, difficult emotions or conflicts with other people, what are my typical ways of dealing with them?

- When I think about these, what are they intended to do?

- What are their unintended consequences?

- How do I acknowledge, face and work on those unintended the consequences from now on?

### EXERCISE 7.3: USING A COMPASSIONATE FORMULATION FORM

This exercise is designed to help you work through the elements of the formulation that we outlined in Figure 7.1, in a similar way as we did for

Alison in Figure 7.2. You can use Worksheet 4 at the end of this chapter to summarize your formulation if you wish.

### Step 1: What are my key threats?

The first step is to identify the things that trigger your threat/protection system. Remember, these may be associated with a range of different emotions, including sadness, anger, disgust, grief etc. Try to think of both situations and events in the past that tended to bring up these emotions, and of situations and events in the present that have the same effects.

Now try to list:
*The past influences on my key threats*

(1)

(2)

(3)

(4)
(and any others . . .)

*The current triggers to my key threats*

(1)

(2)

(3)

(4)
(and any others . . .)

### Step 2: What are my safety strategies?

These are the things that you do, feel or think to help you manage your key threats. They might be directed outwards (external safety strategies), for example, trying to influence other people's judgements of you, or inwards (internal safety strategies), for example, trying to influence your own feelings about yourself and your emotions.

These strategies can be a little tricky to identify at first. The key is to ask yourself what you do, feel or think to protect yourself from re-experiencing things you found distressing in the past, or to avoid painful experiences in the future. It can sometimes be helpful to think about the things other people might notice you do to protect yourself; perhaps you can even talk this through with someone close to you whom you trust to have your best interests at heart.

Now try to list:
*My external safety strategies*

(1)

(2)

(3)

(4)
(and any others . . .)

*My internal safety strategies*

(1)

(2)

(3)

(4)
(and any others . . .)

### Step 3: What are the intended consequences of my safety strategies?
Sometimes we are very aware of the pain and distress that our safety strategies have evolved to help us manage and we use our safety strategies in a very deliberate way. Sometimes, though, these strategies have become more of a habit, with their original purpose lost in the past. Some strategies we will have adopted because we were taught to behave in this way, as a family or social rule passed down to us, and we have no real idea what the strategy is trying to protect us from.

If you do know what you're aiming to achieve or avoid by using a particular safety strategy, it can give you a head start in thinking about alternative ways to cope with the problem. At other times you may need to give up the strategy a little (even if only in your imagination) before you become aware of what it's been doing for you.

You may also find that strategies you have learned, and believe you have needed, actually have no association with your personal threat system when you start to change. This may be particularly true if your safety strategy was 'inherited' from someone else. A good example of this is a rule that 'I need to eat everything on my plate, even if I feel full'. My own grandparents followed this rule, and taught it to us every time they visited. You can see that it was a perfectly understandable safety strategy for ensuring that no food was wasted in a poor family living between the First and Second World Wars, when food supplies were unreliable and the most had to be made of whatever was available. It became nationally important during the Second World War in the UK – with the government reinforcing the message of 'Waste Not Want Not'. It was a less useful eating strategy when I was growing up in the 1960s and 1970s, as my parents (although still working class) were a little more affluent and food supplies were much more readily available, and has the potential unintended consequence of contributing to subsequent generations losing touch with their internal mechanisms for regulating their eating.

If you don't find it easy to work out what the intended consequences of your safety strategies are, it may help to take each of your key threats in turn and try to link it to a particular safety strategy.

Now try to write:

*The intended consequences of each of my safety strategies*

(1)

(2)

(3)

(4)
(and any others . . .)

**Step 4. What are the unintended consequences of my safety strategies?**
As we saw in Alison's story, it is likely that our safety strategies really do help us cope with our key threats – otherwise we would give them up pretty quickly!

Sadly, though, as we have also seen, some of our strategies can have unintended consequences, and these may lead to difficulties later. It is really important to remember that this exercise is designed to help you explore the complexities of your emotional systems and develop greater control over your threat/protection system so that you can beat overeating for good; the idea is *not* to use this new information as a stick to beat yourself with!

As with the previous step, it can be helpful to separate out your safety strategies and to work out the unintended consequences of each of them individually, perhaps with the help of someone else who cares for you.

Now try to write:
*The unintended consequences of my safety strategies*

(1)

(2)

(3)

(4)
(and any others . . .)

Finally, you can explore whether these unintended consequences actually increase the level of threat you experience or mean that you use your safety strategies even more. You may wish to use Worksheet 4 to help you do this. As we saw in Alison's example (Figure 7.2), her unintended consequences led to further problems with assertiveness, comfort eating and dieting.

When you finish this section you can then explore if any of your unintended consequences lead you back into further problems that your eating (or other safety strategies) evolved to help you solve. If they do, you can then draw some lines to represent these connections on Worksheet 4.

## Worksheet 4: My compassionate formulation for overeating

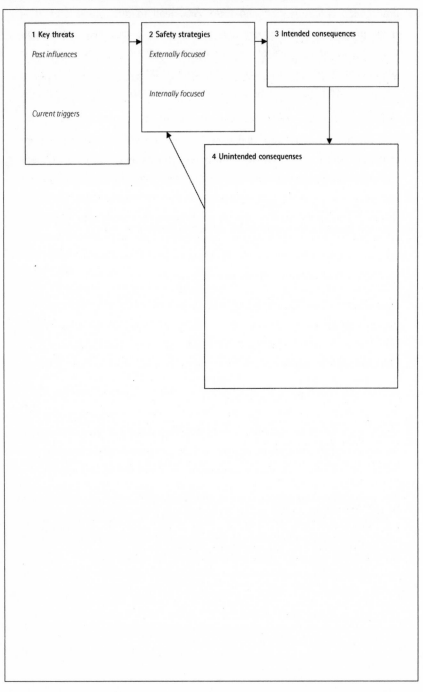

## SUMMARY

In this chapter we have explored a way of making sense of the factors that may have made you likely to overeat in the past and that may keep your overeating going in the present. Using Alison's example, we have also explored how the strategies we use to protect ourselves from unpleasant events or emotions can be helpful to us, but can also have unintended, and sometimes unwanted, consequences. Blaming ourselves for these things can often keep us trapped in a vicious circle of threat and response and can even make things worse. Creating a compassionate formulation for these influences and processes helps us to explore them without blame or criticism so that we can start to think about how to move forward in a more caring, kind and supportive way that takes into account the problems that changing may pose for us.

The chapter has also set out a number of exercises to help you develop your own compassionate formulation for overeating. When you have completed these exercises you can then move on to developing alternative strategies for managing your threat/protection system, and to help with any difficulties that may arise as you give up your old safety strategies. This new and more sensitive way of understanding your relationship with eating will help you to predict the types of problem that you will need help with, and the possible unintended consequences of changing your relationship with food.

In the following chapters we will explore ways of building on this formulation to develop a deeper and more detailed understanding of both the past and present influences on your eating.

# Understanding your current eating pattern

Making sense of your past can help you to make sense of your current relationship with food and to stop criticizing yourself for the way you eat now. It is equally important (and sometimes easier), if you are aiming to stop overeating in the future, to understand your current eating habits and the things that influence you now.

## Using an eating diary

A helpful way to do this is to learn to observe and become mindful of your eating patterns in a structured way by keeping an eating diary. This can be a really helpful tool in changing your relationship with food. So the next part of this chapter will suggest what information you might record and how to make sense of the information you gather. But first it's useful to be clear about the main purposes of learning to monitor your eating habits and the thoughts and emotions that affect them. These are:

- to get an overview of your difficulties;

- to look for and make sense of patterns in triggers to overeating;

- to look for and make sense of things that protect you from overeating;

- to help slow down the 'inevitable' rush to overeat;

- to record your coping thoughts and strategies;

- to record and understand your progress in addressing overeating.

As for how to keep an eating diary, there are only two rules for monitoring your eating:

- Do it in real time – as you eat or as soon as possible afterwards, not at the end of the day.

- Be honest!

**Worksheet 5: Your eating diary**

| Monday 23 March | | | |
|---|---|---|---|
| Situation<br>Where were you?<br>Who were you with?<br>How were you feeling?<br>What were you thinking before you ate? | What you ate or drank (type and amount)<br><br>Physical activity (type and duration) | Overeating?<br>Yes/No | Dieting mindset or comfort food mindset active when eating?<br>Yes/No | Thoughts and feelings<br>These can be thoughts and feelings during or after eating, about doing the diary, or anything else that you think is important |
| | | | | |

The amount of time it takes to get the hang of keeping an eating diary will vary from one person to another, but you'll probably want to spend several weeks or even a few months doing it so that you get a really good overview of your basic eating styles.

Worksheet 5 is a form that you can use to monitor your eating. Take a few moments to read through the headings. It might look a bit daunting at first, so after looking at it section by section we'll go through a real-life example using a day of Alison's diary. (There are a couple of copies of the blank worksheet at the back of the book, and you can take as many more copies of these as you need, or just copy the headings on to fresh sheets of paper.)

## Before eating

The first column is designed to help you make sense of the circumstances that lead up to overeating, or that protect us from either dieting or overeating.

Sometimes overeating can be triggered by being in particular places, or is more common at different times of the year, month or day.

Some people can help us avoid overeating, while others may deliberately or accidentally encourage it. Some of our relationships can be difficult, and our emotions when we're with these people – or after we've been with them – can lead to overeating.

At this point there are two types of feelings we are interested in. The first is your *physical sensations*. These include whether you feel hungry or full, although if you have been dieting or overeating for some time, you may have lost touch with these bodily sensations, so it may not be easy to say at first. You can also record here whether you feel tired, restless, agitated etc.

The other type of feeling we are interested in is your *emotions* – whether you feel anxious, sad, bored, angry, irritable or any of the many other possibilities. You may, of course, be feeling pleasant emotions, such as joy, pleasure or excitement. Usually we will be feeling a mixture of emotions: it is common to feel several emotions at the same time or to have rapid changes in our emotions.

As for what you're thinking at this point, this too may not be easy to pinpoint at first. Sometimes we can be unaware of our thoughts, and it is a skill to be able to recognize them. You may find this easier as you get used to keeping your eating diary. If you do notice you are thinking in a particular way, or about particular things, this can give you a clue to what triggers your eating.

We can break thinking down into three areas:

- memories – positive or unpleasant – that you have before eating;

- thoughts about problems you are facing or going to face in the future;

- thoughts about eating, including the possible benefits of overeating or problems that overeating may create for you.

There may of course be other types of thoughts that you have that are not related to overeating, and again it may be helpful to write these down too.

## What you eat and/or drink, and what physical activity you take

In the second column you can write what you are eating or drinking. Ideally you will also record roughly how much you have eaten – however, don't worry about recording or adding up calories at this point. You will only do this when you review your diary, and we'll explore how to do this a little later in the chapter. This column will be very helpful later on when you are working out whether your overeating is actually related to your not giving your body enough food during the day. It may also help you notice whether any particular types of food are more likely to be associated with overeating. Remember that there are a number of 'non-foods' that are also associated with overeating. These include alcohol, medications and some illegal drugs. It is also important to list what and how much of these you take every day to help you work out if they affect how much you eat.

It is also useful to keep a brief note of the types and amount of physical activity that you do: for example, noting down if you do an hour of housework, or go to the gym for thirty minutes each day. The information in this column can help you to work out your energy and nutritional balance, and notice whether particular types of food trigger overeating.

## Have you overeaten?

The third column asks you if you believe that you have overeaten. This is important, because sometimes we think that we have or haven't overeaten because of the types of food we eat or our feelings at the time, rather than as a result of an objective decision about what our body needed at a particular time, or how our eating compares to that of people who are more in touch with their bodies' needs and appetites.

## What mindset are you in while you are eating?

The fourth column prompts you to consider what kind of mindset you are in when you are eating. This will help you to recognize what kind of eating you're doing and also to think about what problems this mindset is trying to help you manage. The main types of mindset we are interested in here are the ones that are most likely to influence your eating – the 'comfort food' and 'dieting' mindsets. However, you may also find that other types of mindset, such as being in an anxious, depressed or angry state of mind, can also influence your overeating.

## What are you thinking and feeling?

The final column explores your thoughts and feelings while you're eating and afterwards. In a more advanced version of this diary you can also use this column to record thoughts, feelings or things you do that help you manage your urges to overeat or limit overeating. In your early diaries you may find that you have a lot of self-critical thoughts and feelings about overeating, or find that overeating helps you to manage some difficult thoughts or feelings.

In Figure 8.1 you can see one day of Alison's completed diary.

As with all the exercises in this chapter, it's important that you set about keeping the diary at your own pace. To begin with, it may be easier just to record what you eat, the time of day and who you are with. When you are used to doing, this you can then start to include your feelings and thoughts before and after eating. You can leave it until you feel fairly used to doing this before you try decide whether you actually overate and whether you were in a 'dieting' or 'comfort food' mindset before, during or after eating.

## Blocks to monitoring

Monitoring may look like a pretty simple exercise – after all, it only has two rules: complete it in real time, and be honest! In practice, however, many people find they come up against obstacles when they start trying to monitor their eating. These blocks generally fall into one of two categories: practical and emotional.

Practical blocks to monitoring include:

- difficulty in learning to use the form;

- difficulty in keeping the diary private;

- problems completing it when other people are around;

- finding the time to do it.

Emotional blocks to monitoring include:

- resenting doing the task;

- worrying that being more observant and mindful of your difficulties will make your eating or feelings worse;

- seeing what you eat written down making you feel more self-critical or ashamed;

- worrying about what others will think if they see you doing the diary.

It is helpful to identify any of your own blocks to monitoring, and to try to find solutions to them, before you begin to keep your diary. Worksheet 6

| Monday 23 March | | | | |
|---|---|---|---|---|
| Situation<br>Where were you?<br>Who were you with?<br>How were you feeling?<br>What were you thinking before you ate? | What you ate or drank (type and amount)<br>Physical activity (type and duration) | Overeating?<br>Yes/No | Dieting mindset or comfort food mindset active when eating?<br>Yes/No | Thoughts and feelings<br>These can be thoughts and feelings during or after eating, about doing the diary, or anything else that you think is important |
| 8 a.m., at home, alone<br>A bit hungry, tired<br>Not really thinking about anything | Cereal, 2 slices of toast, tea | No | No | Felt OK about eating, a bit worried about going to work today |
| 10 a.m., at work, with colleagues<br>A bit anxious<br>Worried about difficult meeting later today | Tea and 5 ginger biscuits | Yes | Comfort food | Felt a little worried that colleagues would think I was greedy, but felt I needed the food to calm me down |
| 12.30 p.m., at work, alone<br>A bit queasy, not hungry<br>More anxious about meeting | Tea and 10 more biscuits<br>Had planned to have lunch but couldn't face it | Maybe? | Comfort, but also thought I would cut back on the biscuits for the rest of the week | Felt greedy |

| | | | | |
|---|---|---|---|---|
| 1.45 p.m. at restaurant, alone Very upset by meeting, felt angry with boss and useless Mainly thinking about meeting and worried about what other people thought about me | Burger meal, large milkshake | No | Mainly comfort but planned not to eat for the rest of the day | Felt OK about eating, but very down about myself, worried about going back to work |
| 10.30 p.m. home, with partner Still upset about work Felt I deserved a treat | 4 glasses of wine, takeaway meal, plus leftovers Individual tub of ice cream | Yes | Dieting mind until just before the meal, but partner came in from work late and brought in a takeaway | Didn't want to eat, but when I did felt out of control and could not stop Felt angry with myself for overeating, planning to eat a lot less tomorrow |

**Figure 8.1:** Alison's eating diary

is a form you can use to help you do this – or you can of course create your own. Figure 8.2 shows a worked example of the form.

## Managing emotional blocks to monitoring

Practical blocks sound easier to address, but in fact are often easier to manage once you have worked though emotional blocks. So let's start with some of the most common of these.

The first emotional block for most people is finding a reason for keeping the diary that will prompt you to fill it in even if it is a struggle. We will explore motivation to change in Chapter 10, but for now you might try thinking of keeping a diary as a leap of faith – something that's worth a try to see if it can help you. Again, you may wish to explore the idea of keeping a diary from the perspective of your compassionate image. What would 'you at your best' or your compassionate companion say to help you take this leap of faith? How would they express their understanding of and care for your real and honest concerns that the diary could be emotionally challenging for you? What would they say about the advantages of keeping a diary for you personally? What kind of compassionate plan might they come up with to help you deal with your emotional blocks?

Many people worry that doing the diary will be upsetting. Well, this can happen, particularly as you begin to make connections between eating and your thoughts and feelings. However, this distress tends to be temporary and it can help to remind you that what you're doing has a purpose: that if you can learn to tolerate a certain amount of distress now, you're likely to be better able to prevent yourself overeating in the future, and to learn new ways to manage your thoughts and feelings. Even so, keeping the diary short, not re-reading it at the end of the day, or even keeping each eating episode written in a separate place (so you don't have to see your day's eating all in one go) can help you to avoid getting upset. You may also wish to plan soothing and distraction exercises to do after you have written your diary. By using whichever of these techniques suits you, you can put together a plan for making your diary emotionally manageable.

**Worksheet 6: Managing blocks to monitoring**

| My personal blocks | Compassionate things I can say to myself or do to get past the block |
| --- | --- |
| | |

| My personal blocks | Compassionate things I can say to myself or do to get past the block |
| --- | --- |
| It brings attention to my overeating | It's understandable to feel a bit upset when I become aware of the difficulties – but in my heart I would like to move forward on this and so learning how to face my embarrassment or distress can be helpful in the long run. Maybe I can try it a few times and see how it goes. |
| This is boring and I really don't like having to do these kinds of monitoring things | It's true, this can be boring, but maybe I could just have a couple of tries to get going and see how I do. Perhaps I could put a small note on the fridge to remind myself. To be honest, there are lots of things I do in my life that I find it boring, so this doesn't have to be a block. I am quite capable of doing boring things if I recognize they can be helpful in the long run. |
| I guess I feel bad because I'm being quite critical really – I don't like myself because of my overeating | I should remember that this is not my fault. I have a see-food-and-eat-it brain – and the food industry has encouraged me to want certain foods. I also learned to use eating to support myself emotionally because it helped at the time. It's more important to be kind and understanding and recognize that there is a problem here and that if I go gently and kindly with myself I can begin to find new ways forward. |

**Figure 8.2:** Managing blocks to monitoring: an example

It's also important to make sure you tackle your diary from a compassionate mindset. Diaries can often be used by people who diet or overeat as a way of beating themselves up for what they have eaten or why they eat – and this is absolutely *not* the idea here. Remember all that we discovered in the earlier chapters of this book about where our impulses and habits to do with eating come from, way back in our common ancestry and also in our early personal histories. The habits and practices you've been using are just the best ways you've found so far to deal with your own circumstances; what we're aiming to do now is to give you new and better ways to do this with information and understanding that you haven't had before.

## Managing practical blocks to monitoring

The eating diary form set out in Worksheet 5 may look a bit cumbersome; still, many people get used to it fairly quickly and become happy to fill it in using this format. However, this is certainly not the only way to do it. Several people I have worked with prefer to keep the information in their own personal diaries; this can help the task to feel more private and special to you. By all means buy yourself a nice diary or notebook, ideally one that can be locked or is inconspicuous, to use as your monitoring record.

I have found that people can be really ingenious in managing this task. For example, texting the information to one's own mobile phone can be a good way both to get the information down quickly and to keep it private.

As for the time it takes, monitoring is designed to be done quite rapidly – I would suggest taking no more than a minute or so for each episode of eating. So it shouldn't take any more than ten to fifteen minutes a day. It is important, however, not to leave this until the end of the day and do it all at once then. It really does help to have the information recorded at the time you're eating, or at least immediately afterwards. Most people can remember what they ate and when at the end of the day, but it's not so easy to remember accurately how you were feeling and what you were thinking at the time. You might want to use a personal code to note down your feelings and thoughts: like texting, this can be a good way to get the information down privately and quickly. Other ways of doing this are to record a few short lines as a phone message or email, or on a scrap of paper. It doesn't matter how you get the information down, really, so long as you do it as soon as possible. If you end up with a collection of what seem like scrappy notes, you can always write up a 'neat' copy at the end of the day. A word of warning here, though: I suggest you try to do this fairly rapidly, as dwelling for too long on a whole day's eating, feelings and thoughts might leave you feeling a bit upset or uncomfortable.

## Using your diary to make sense of your eating

Once you've got used to keeping your eating diary, you can start using the diary review sheet provided as Worksheet 7 to help you draw together the information you've collected and start to identify the things that protect you from, as well as those that put you at risk of, overeating. Again, it is important when you set about reviewing your diary that you do so from the perspective of your compassionate mind, exploring the patterns you find in a genuine spirit of concerned curiosity, wanting to understand and then find ways to alleviate the uncomfortable and perhaps painful emotions that your overeating both helps you with and causes for you. It's also a good idea to plan to set aside time to soothe any distress the reviewing process causes.

When I review diaries with my clients, we put aside at least an hour or so at the end of the week and review a whole week's worth of diaries. This gives us a much better idea of patterns; indeed, sometimes we will review four weeks' worth of diaries together to get a longer-term perspective. It can take a week or two to get the hang of keeping the diary, so you might want to wait until you feel you have a week's worth of complete daily records before you can start your review.

As we have seen in previous chapters, there are a whole range of factors that can affect your eating habits. When we are reviewing a diary we aim to cover as many of these as possible. They include the following.

## Eating pattern

As we found in Chapter 3, eating patterns can significantly affect our risk of overeating. When looking at your diary it is important to look for the spaces between eating episodes. Your body can last for about three or for hours before it starts getting hungry. Eating more frequently than this can put us out of touch with our hunger; leaving longer gaps puts us at risk of overeating at the next meal.

## Energy balance

As we saw in Chapter 2, our bodies need a certain amount of energy every day just to keep our physical systems going; and we need a variable amount on top of this to fuel whatever we do during the day. If we overeat we can lose touch with our bodily needs; if, on the other hand, we are trying to eat less than our body needs we are likely to overeat – as well as to experience a range of psychological and physical side-effects. So what we're aiming at is an 'energy balance' – eating just the right amount to support our physical systems and our activities.

Many people who overeat will be quite good at estimating their energy intake (in the form of calories), although they may be less aware of the amount of energy they use or need. Unless you have access to a dietitian who can work this out for you, this is a skill that you will need to develop. We'll explore how to do this in more detail in Chapter 11, but it's worth taking a look at the basic principles here.

The easiest (but by no means easy way) of estimating your energy intake is to become familiar with the calorie content of what you eat and drink. There are many commercial calorie-counting books and websites that can help you to do this. Again, you might find adding up your calorie intake an uncomfortable exercise at first; try to view it as a necessary step in helping you to gain control over your eating and support yourself compassionately while you do it.

Ideally you are aiming for an energy intake of 2,000 calories per day if you are a woman and 2,500 calories if you are a man. It is normal to have a variation of about 200 calories a day – your body is more than capable of adjusting to this – but your overall aim is a balance in your energy over the week, which means an energy consumption of around 14,000 calories per week if you are a woman, 17,500 if you are a man.

Keeping an eye on your calorie intake to try to establish an appropriate energy balance can really help you to tackle overeating. It is likely that if you are using this book to help you beat overeating you may find it difficult to balance your energy at this stage. Don't worry; we will work on how to do this in more detail in Chapter 11.

## What you eat and drink

Many people find that specific types of food act as a trigger to overeating. These may be foods that we associate with comfort, or that are usually 'forbidden' in some way, or simply foods that we really like! Learning to eat and enjoy these types of food in moderation can be really important in managing overeating.

## Times, people, places

Often overeating happens in a regular or predictable way: for example, many of us overeat at weekends, or when we are with others who overeat. Understanding these patterns can help us plan to manage these situations in another way.

## Your feelings and overeating

As we explored earlier, it can be helpful to divide feelings into *physical sensations* (including hunger) and *emotions* (such as anger, boredom or anxiety), although of course our physical sensations and emotions are often mingled together. It can sometimes be difficult to identify both kinds of feeling, particularly if eating helps you to manage them. Sometimes you may have to delay responding to the urge to overeat for a little while to be able to identify your feelings more clearly. We will explore how to do this in Chapter 12. Once you can identify these feelings, you are on your way to learning to understand and manage them in a more compassionate way.

## Your thoughts and overeating

There are many ways in which our thoughts can lead to overeating. They can:

- give us positive permission to overeat, telling us for example that we 'deserve food' because we have been good or had a hard time;

- allow us to punish ourselves with food;

- encourage us to hope that eating will help us to manage unpleasant feelings or experiences;

- encourage, support or bully us into dieting, and thus increase our risk of overeating later;

- provide rules that lead to accidental or habitual overeating (such as 'I must always clear my plate').

Our thoughts are also very likely to be intertwined with our feelings. Sometimes our thoughts have less to with eating itself than with how we think about ourselves, or how we think other people will think about us after we have overeaten, or if they find out that we overeat. As we have seen, these patterns can lead us into vicious cycles of secret eating or dieting to deal with the painful feelings that this type of self-criticism and shame can lead to.

All of these ways of thinking are understandable and very common, and it is important to understand and be compassionate with the way that these thoughts develop.

Our thoughts can also help us to manage our urges to overeat or to cope when we have overeaten. Recognizing, supporting and encouraging the thoughts that can help us to manage overeating is a major step in controlling overeating. Your diary can help you to identify and build upon these thoughts, and to develop new ones.

One cautionary note: I encourage my clients not to review their diary if they have had a particularly difficult day, nor to do it just before they go to bed, when they will probably be tired and may be tempted to brood critically on what they have recorded rather than analyse it compassionately. It is better to do the review when we are feeling relatively calm and alert and able to learn from our diaries.

## Making sense of Alison's diary

In the final section of this chapter we will review the sample day of Alison's diary shown as Figure 8.1 to give you an idea of how reviewing a diary works in practice, and how what you learn can help you to beat overeating for good.

As I mentioned earlier, usually the more information we have the easier it is to make sense of a diary, so it's a good idea to review a whole week's

**Worksheet 7: Diary review sheet**

---

Eating pattern
How long do I leave between eating episodes?                                    _____ hours
How many times per day do I eat more often than every 3–4
hours?                                                                                                     _____
How many times do I eat less often than every 3–4 hours?             _____

Energy needs
What is my daily energy need?                                                       _____ calories
How much energy do I take in each day?                                       _____ calories
How much energy do I use up each day?                                       _____ calories
Am I eating more or less than I need each day?                              More/Less

What I eat and drink
Are there specific types of food that trigger overeating?

Are there any foods that help me not to overeat?

Are there any things I take into my body that affect my appetite (e.g. medication, drugs, alcohol)?

Times, people, places
Are there any times, people or places that make overeating more likely?

Are there any times, people or places that protect me from overeating?

My feelings and overeating
Are there any feelings that make my overeating worse?

Are these physical sensations, such as hunger?

Are these emotions, such as sadness, boredom, anger, anxiety?

My thoughts and overeating
Am I in a dieting mindset before, during or after overeating?              Yes/No
Am I in a comfort food mindset before, during or after overeating?     Yes/No
Do I give myself permission to overeat as a treat?                              Yes/No
Do I use overeating to punish myself?                                               Yes/No
Do I hope that overeating will help me manage difficult feelings, memories,
or events?                                                                                         Yes/No
Do I follow certain rules or habits that I have been taught about eating?  Yes/No
Do I criticize or bully myself about what I have eaten or the way that I eat?  Yes/No
Am I worried about what other people will think about my overeating?    Yes/No

*If you answer 'yes' to any of these questions, try to be as specific as you can about exactly what you are thinking and, if you can, where you learned to think in this way.*

records together. There may also be monthly or seasonal patterns to our relationship with overeating that we only see when we look at a sequence of diary records over a much longer period. However, even looking at one day can be very revealing – and that's what we're going to do here.

When we review Alison's diary we see that four of her eating episodes occurred relatively close together (at 8 a.m., 10 a.m., 12.30 p.m. and 1.45 p.m.) but that there was then a very long gap until her final meal of the day at 10.30 p.m. On reflection she noticed that she wasn't particularly hungry at 10 a.m. or 12.30 p.m., but in the evening had been fending off feeling hungry from about 6 p.m. By looking over a lot of similar days' records, Alison became aware of a couple of issues that she decided to work on. The first was learning to eat when her body was more likely to be hungry and to avoid eating when she didn't need to, even if that meant not eating at times when other people were. The second one, which was related to the first, was a longstanding pattern of trying not to eat in the evening – which in fact amounted to a 'rule' that she should not eat at this time of day. This left her feeling deprived, hungry and likely to overeat if she did break her rule.

Alison also noticed that other people being around and being on her own both increased her risk of overeating in different ways. She found it hard not to overeat when she was with work colleagues, or if her partner offered her food to cheer her up. However, when she was alone she also tended to comfort eat. Alison was able to identify both anxiety and anger as feelings that she managed by using food.

Before starting to keep a diary Alison believed that she overate all of the time. She was surprised to find that some of her meals (e.g. breakfast) were actually normal portions. Later on, when she worked out her energy intake for this day, she found that she had eaten at least 1,500 calories more than her body needed. This wasn't really news to Alison, although she did find it upsetting to see it written down. What was more interesting was that at lunchtime she couldn't face eating the sandwich, bag of crisps and apple she'd taken to work because it felt like overeating – but that actually these added up to fewer calories than the biscuits that she ate because she didn't want to overeat.

As she thought more about what she'd eaten on this day, Alison remembered that she had always been offered biscuits to help her manage being upset when she was growing up. This helped her to think about the urge to eat biscuits being a good warning sign that she might need to deal with her feelings, as well as to focus on eating foods that would be more filling, like her sandwich and crisps (even if they felt too fattening), to help her avoid overeating later.

The final thing that Alison realized about what she was eating and drinking was that alcohol tended to make her feel hungrier and less able to control her urges to overeat. This helped her to think about changing her drinking habits, and in particular trying to reduce the amount of alcohol she drank if she was upset, anxious or angry.

Alison was particularly skilled in recognizing the types of mindset she was in when she was eating. She fluctuated between her 'comfort food' and her 'dieting' mindsets. She noticed that these mindsets often clouded her whole day, but also helped her to deal with threatening events – for example, the distressing meeting she had at work on this day. Thinking about food in one way or another helped her to avoid thinking about the meeting for large parts of the day. She was also able to notice that she often struggled with feeling greedy after eating, became worried about what other people thought about her if they saw her eating, and could get very angry with herself when she overate. She noticed that her anger was helpful in fuelling her urges to diet and to avoid being seen as greedy, and preventing her from overeating later, but often led to her feeling even worse and needing to comfort eat to manage this.

It took Alison several weeks of diary-keeping to identify these patterns clearly, and some time after that to decide which areas to work on first in trying gradually to reduce her overeating. In the next chapter we will explore how you can use the information from your diary to develop a compassionate understanding of your own difficulties and to set realistic goals for addressing your overeating.

**SUMMARY**

This chapter has explored a practical way of recording and exploring the current patterns and triggers than may influence your eating habits now. In the next chapter we will put this information together to help you develop a personal understanding of your eating and how your eating habits help you to manage your threat system. We will also explore how to put all of this information together by revisiting the compassionate formulation for your overeating.

# 9 How does your overeating work now?

In the previous chapter we explored how keeping an eating diary can help you to become more observant of your overeating, and how you can begin to make sense of the information you gather in this way by reviewing your diary. Now, drawing on both that chapter and Chapter 7, in which we explored how both events in the past and things you are dealing with in the present can affect how and what you eat, we will work on putting all this information together to see how you may have been using overeating to help manage your very complex emotional system and 'see-food-and-eat it' brain.

It's worth pausing here to repeat that if you're struggling to deal with overeating you are certainly not alone: overeating is a problem for over half of the Western world. Nor does it mean that there is anything wrong with *you*. Overeating is likely to be the outcome of the complex interactions between your genetic makeup, biological mechanisms that helped us all successfully survive famine, and events in your own life that have either taught you to overeat or taught you that overeating could help you in some way.

In the first three chapters of this book we explored these mechanisms in some detail and introduced the 'three systems' approach to understanding how we regulate our emotions. In Chapter 7 we introduced the idea of a 'compassionate formulation' for overeating. We are now going to revisit all these ideas and draw them together to help you construct a new and more developed formulation for your difficulties with overeating.

## Overeating and the 'three systems' of emotional regulation

The 'three systems' model of emotional regulation can be a very helpful way of thinking about the ways in which our overeating can be used (deliberately or accidentally) to manage our emotional life, and to think about how overeating can affect our emotional life.

As you may remember, we are interested in three main systems:

- the threat/protection system, which is mainly about helping to stop us doing, or get us away from, things that we believe are unpleasant or dangerous to us;

- the drive/achievement system, which is concerned with helping us reach specific goals;

- the affiliative contentment/soothing system, which focuses on making us feel calm, soothed and cared for.

We need all three systems to help us manage the challenges of life; and all three of them can be affected by, and can in turn affect, the eating habits we learn and get used to. As we have seen, feeling soothed by food ('the comfort food mind') can replace other ways of feeling cared for, soothed and contented. The 'dieting mind' is often connected with the drive/ achievement system, so that we feel that dieting can both be an achieve-ment in itself and also help us get closer to other goals we have in life. Both the 'comfort food' and 'dieting' minds can be turned on when we feel under threat in some way. These threats can be either external (things that are happening to us) or internal (from our memories, thoughts and feelings). Often a threat has elements of both types. Once our threat/ protection system is active, we tend to see things that we would normally feel OK about as threats too. Do remember, by the way, that this rapid escalation of the threat/protection system is perfectly normal: after all, it evolved to protect us, and it wouldn't have been much good at that if it had been easy to ignore! But because this system is so active and so powerful, it can quickly become difficult for us to see the wood for the trees, so to speak, as we seem to be surrounded by threats and under pressure to respond to or retreat from them. So it can be helpful to work out in advance what things trigger the system, and then what additional issues arise once it has got into its stride.

In a compassionate mind approach to overeating, we are particularly interested in helping you work out whether the balance between these three systems has become skewed. We also want to see if 'comfort food' or 'dieting' or other overeating mindsets (e.g. 'eating for fun' or 'eating to belong') have got entangled with these systems. Finally, we want to see if the ways you have been using to try to manage these systems have had unintentional side-effects that are making it even more difficult for you to manage your emotions.

## How overeating may help us manage emotions

In the next section of this chapter we will explore how overeating may help you to manage your three emotional regulation systems. This analysis, involving a series of key questions, will provide you with a deeper understanding of how eating helps you in the here and now. Combined with the information you began to gather in Chapter 7 about past and present influences on your eating habits and why you may be sensitive to particular types of threat, it will give you the basis for a new personal compassionate formulation for overeating.

This analysis revolves around nine questions that help us to make sense of the reasons why we overeat and the unintended consequences of overeating. Here they are:

(1) Am I at greater risk of overeating when my threat/protection system comes into play?

(2) What types of threat are most likely to trigger my overeating?

(3) Are there any other threats that I pay attention to once my threat/protection mindset is active?

(4) How does eating help me to cope when my threat/protection system is switched on?

(5) Does eating help me to feel soothed?

(6) Does eating help me turn off or tone down the threat/protection system?

(7)  Does eating activate my drive/achievement system?

(8)  How do I hope that eating will make me feel safer (the intended consequence of eating)?

(9)  What are the unintended consequences of overeating?

We will work through these nine questions, using Alison's thoughts and responses, to show you how they can help guide your exploration, before you have a go at analysing how your three systems relate to your own overeating habits.

## Alison's analysis of eating and the three systems

Using her first 'compassionate formulation for overeating', which we saw in Chapter 7, and the completed pages of her eating diary (one of which we looked at in Chapter 8), Alison began to develop her analysis of how her overeating related to her three emotional systems, taking the nine key questions in turn – sometimes singly and sometimes in groups, starting with the first three questions.

## Key question

(1)  Am I at greater risk of overeating when my threat/protection system comes into play?

(2)  What types of threat are most likely to trigger my overeating?

(3)  Are there any other threats that I pay attention to once my threat/protection mindset is active?

Alison noticed that the biggest trigger to overeating on the day she completed her diary was the meeting just before lunchtime with her boss. This was a routine meeting to review her work performance. Alison wanted to use it to make her boss aware that she had taken on a lot of work recently that was beyond both her pay grade and her training. She had spent a lot of time planning how to let her boss know that she was upset about this additional burden and wanted them to reduce the demands made on her. However, Alison had found it difficult to be assertive with her employers in the past and already expected that, even if she told them about the problem, they would do nothing to rectify the situation. Alison recognized that her problems with assertiveness cropped up in many relationships and believed that they dated back to her childhood. She noticed that both anticipated and actual experiences of wanting to be assertive with others tended to activate her threat/protection system.

Alison also noticed that when her threat/protection system was in play she was likely to remember times in her life when her needs had not been met by others. She was also likely to be angry with herself for finding it difficult to be assertive.

## Key questions

(4)  How does eating help me to cope when my threat/protection system is switched on?

(5)  Does eating help me to feel soothed?

(6)  Does eating help me turn off or tone down the threat/protection system?

Alison noticed that eating helped her to deal with feelings of anxiety about the meeting in several ways. First, the food helped to soothe her anxiety. She also noticed that the types of food she ate reminded her of people who had cared for her. For example, the smell of the ginger biscuits she ate at 10 a.m. reminded her of her grandmother, who used to bake with her when she was growing up.

Alison also found that focusing on the taste and pleasure of eating her burger helped to take her mind off the meeting after it happened. It also temporarily distracted her from self-critical thoughts about her performance in the meeting.

## Key question

(7)  Does eating activate my drive/achievement system?

Some people who overeat are proud of their ability to eat more than others. There are even world records for the most hot dogs you can eat! However, for most people this is not the way their achievement system is activated when they overeat. More usually, it is either anticipation of the pleasure of eating or planning to diet that will activate the drive/achievement system.

Alison had both of these experiences. She had not planned to have a burger and milkshake for lunch that day – indeed, she had actually brought her sandwich lunch to work. But once the meeting was over she told herself that she deserved something nice to eat because she had survived what she thought would be a very difficult meeting (in fact her boss praised some of her work and was not as critical as she had predicted). She spent the hour between finishing the meeting and her lunch break anticipating the flavours of her favourite food and the pleasure it would bring her.

Once she had finished eating her burger, she then spent a lot of time thinking about how she needed to diet to manage the extra food she had eaten that day. She remembered the times she had dieted and lost a little weight in the past, and the sense of achievement that eating less would bring her.

As we can see, the drive/achievement system can be turned on by the things we actually do, but a lot of the time the focus is on how we will feel when we have achieved our goals: to this extent the drive/achievement system can often be driven as much by hope and wanting as by actually getting what we want.

## Key question

(8)  How do I hope that eating will make me feel safer? (The intended consequences of overeating.)

Alison hoped that eating would both calm her anxiety and reward her for facing a difficult situation. She gave herself permission to overeat by telling herself that she would diet later. Planning her diet also helped reduce her anxiety and manage her self-criticism by giving her something else to focus on. She also hoped that dieting would make her happier in the longer term, particularly as it helped to boost her self-confidence.

## Key question

(9) What are the unintended consequences of overeating?

This question took Alison a little more time to explore. She noticed that although eating did help her feel a little less anxious, after overeating she often felt greedy and out of control (i.e. self-critical). She worried that other people would also think she was greedy and out of control. Alison was worried about the effect of overeating on her health, but this concern tended to be less important than managing her fear of being criticized when her threat/protection system was more active.

On further reflection, Alison noticed that although eating helped her to reduce her anxiety before the meeting, it meant that she had given less thought to how she was going to be assertive with her boss, or to addressing this very important issue in her life in the longer term. And after the meeting, her focus on rewarding herself with food for surviving the encounter meant that she didn't really compassionately listen to her sadness for the impact that not being assertive had had on her life, or make sense of her anger and grief for having her needs ignored for so long.

## *Your own analysis of eating and the three systems*

Having read Alison's analysis of how her eating related to her emotional systems, you may now wish to develop your own. You can use the information you have gathered from your diary and the first draft of your compassionate formulation from Chapter 7, as well as any other observations you (or other people) have made about your eating, to help you answer the nine questions.

The nine key questions are set out below with some brief comments that may help you answer them, and again in Worksheet 8 with space for your answers. Before you set about trying to write down your answers, once again spend a few moments slowing your breathing and bringing to mind your compassionate sense of self so that you are looking at these questions from a compassionate frame of mind, with a genuine curiosity based on a desire to understand in order to be helpful – not critical. Now spend some time writing out your own thoughts on each of the questions.

(1) *Am I at greater risk of overeating when my threat/protection system comes on line?*
   If so, what ideas do you have about why this might happen?

(2) *What types of threats are most likely to trigger my overeating?*
   Try to think about what reasons there may be for this, perhaps by thinking about your personal history or current circumstances.

(3) *Are there any other threats that I pay attention to once my threat/protection mindset is online?*
   Often when our threat system comes online we can end up in threat spirals, feeling more and more threatened. This type of threat escalation is very normal. It can be useful to identify any new types of threats that emerge and how your eating may help you deal with them as well as with the original threat that was triggered.

(4) *How does eating help me to cope when my threat/protection system comes online?*

(5) *Does eating help me to feel soothed?*
   If you feel it does, think about in what way it does this; for example, does it help you to feel numb, bring in other soothing memories, etc.?

(6) *Does eating help me turn off or tone down the threat/protection system?*

(7) *Does eating activate my drive/achievement system?*
   For example, is it linked to having fun, or does compensating for overeating by dieting give you a feeling of pride, achievement and being in control?

(8) *How do I hope that eating will make me feel safer?*
What are the intended consequences of overeating for you?

(9) *What are the unintended consequences of overeating?*

Sometimes it is helpful to do several separate analyses, to help us explore the different threats that overeating helps us with. For example, Alison could have worked through one to help her explore her feelings of being criticized by people she worked with, and another to explore concerns she had about upsetting other people in her life. If there were any differences between the two analyses, this might have suggested approaches she could take to managing the key threats she experienced and the safety strategies she used.

## Putting it all together: a new compassionate formulation for your overeating

In Chapter 7 we introduced the idea of a 'compassionate formulation' to help you make sense of your overeating. Building on this with the work we have done Chapter 8 and so far in this chapter, you can now put together the information you have gathered about your history and your current eating habits, and the analysis of how your eating habits relate to your three emotional systems, to generate an overview of why your overeating developed, how it may be helping you now, and how the unintended consequences of eating may trap you in cycles of overeating that can be very difficult to escape.

As you may recall, the compassionate formulation is made up of four elements:

- key threats, and the past and present influences that activate them;

- safety strategies, which can be used to provide us with a sense of external or internal safety;

- intended consequences of our safety strategies;

- unintended consequences of our safety strategies.

**Worksheet 8: Nine key questions for analysing the relationship between eating and the three emotional systems**

1   Am I at greater risk of overeating when my threat/protection system comes into play?

2   What types of threat are most likely to trigger my overeating?

3   Are there any other threats that I pay attention to once my threat/protection mindset is active?

4   How does eating help me to cope when my threat/protection system is switched on?

5   Does eating help me to feel soothed?

6   Does eating help me turn off or tone down the threat/protection system?

7   Does eating activate my drive/achievement system?

8   How do I hope that eating will make me feel safer?

9   What are the unintended consequences of overeating?

We are also interested in how the unintended consequences of our safety strategies can lead to further difficulties that we end up using our safety strategies to solve, setting up vicious circles.

It is important to remember that our formulation is always a 'best guess' at explaining our eating habits. As you get to understand your overeating better, you can always update your formulation by adding new things or taking bits out.

Exercise 9.1 takes you through the same four steps to construct a new compassionate formulation for overeating. Just as you did the first time around, take your time with this. Work at a pace you can manage, and always bring your compassionate image into mind before you attempt to answer the questions. You can use Worksheet 9 to record your formulation as you build it up.

If you find you are becoming self-critical or that the exercise is too much for you to manage, step away from the exercise and, before you go any further, bring your compassionate mind into play again, using your soothing breathing rhythm or safe place image, and spend some time focusing on your compassionate image.

### EXERCISE 9.1: DRAWING UP A NEW COMPASSIONATE FORMULATION FOR YOUR OVEREATING

#### Step 1: What are my key threats?

This is where you identify the things that trigger your threat/protection system. Remember, these may involve a range of different emotions, for example sadness, anger, disgust or grief. You may find it helpful to use the notes you have made about your personal history and your eating diary to identify times when you have had to deal with events and emotions that you have found difficult. You can then look for patterns and triggers to your threat/protection system.

Now try to list:
*The past influences on my key threats*

(1)

## Worksheet 9: My new compassionate formulation for overeating

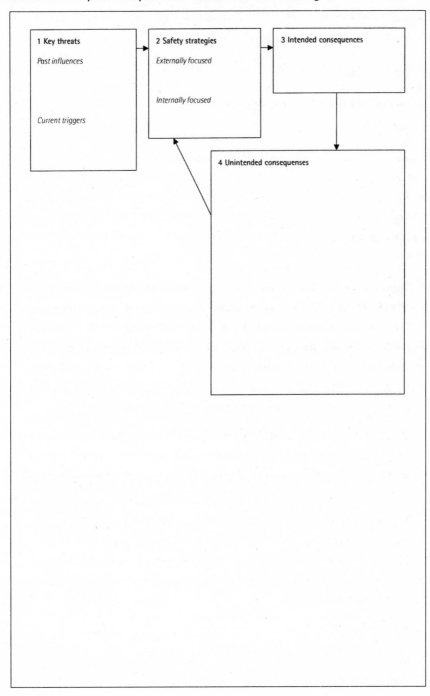

(2)

(3)

(4)
(and any others . . .)

*The current triggers to my key threats*

(1)

(2)

(3)

(4)
(and any others . . .)

### Step 2: What are my safety strategies?

These are the things that you do, feel or think to help you manage your key threats. Alison's example mainly explored her behavioural safety strategies: trying to please others, comfort eating and dieting. Other strategies can include thoughts that protect you from powerful emotions, such as not allowing yourself to get close to others, or always blaming yourself when things go wrong. They can also include habitual emotional reactions, such as disgust, to keep us away from things we find threatening.

If you find it difficult to identify these thoughts and emotions, it may be helpful to consider what other people might notice that you do to protect yourself; you might perhaps be able to talk this over with someone whom you trust.

Now try to list:
*My safety strategies*

(1)

(2)

(3)

(4)
(and any others . . .)

**Step 3: What are the intended consequences of my safety strategies?**
We may use our safety strategies in a very deliberate way, or we may find that these strategies have become something of a habit, with their original purpose lost in the past.

Knowing what you aim to achieve or avoid by using a particular safety strategy makes it easier to start thinking about alternative ways to cope with the problem. However, sometimes you may need actually to give up the strategy a little before you become aware of the role that it has been playing, and so be able to start considering other ways to perform the same function.

You might find that working on your key threats individually, linking each of them to a safety strategy, helps you to work out what the intended consequences of each of your safety strategies is.

Now try to list:
*The intended consequences for each of my safety strategies*

(1)

(2)

(3)

(4)
(and any others . . .)

**Step 4: What are the unintended consequences of my safety strategies?**
We have now seen some of the unintended consequences of our strategies that can lead to further difficulties. It can be helpful to work on each strategy separately, using your personal history, your diaries, your own wisdom and the helpful observations of others who care for you to work out the unintended consequences of your own safety strategies.

Now try to list:
*The unintended consequences of my safety strategies*

(1)

(2)

(3)

(4)
(and any others . . .)

Finally, you can explore whether these unintended consequences actually increase the level of threat you feel or encourage you to intensify your safety strategies.

Once you have completed your formulation, you are then in a position to start developing alternative strategies to managing your threat/protection system. Your new understanding of your relationship with eating will help you to predict the types of problem that you will need help with, and the possible unintended consequences of changing your relationship with food. In the next chapter we will explore how we how we can use this new understanding to motivate you to make changes in your eating.

### SUMMARY

In this chapter we have worked on expanding your personal formulation to explore the ways in which it may help you to manage key threats that have arisen from your past or present experiences by exploring how your eating works now. Although it can be a little daunting at first, learning to use and analyse your diary can be a valuable way of recording your 'here and now' relationship with eating. It can help you to identify a wide range of influences on your eating and will be the basis for your plan to overcome overeating, which we will explore in the final chapters of this book.

# 10 Motivating yourself to change

In this chapter we will explore a way of understanding how the process of changing our behaviour, thoughts and feelings works. If you are reading this book it is likely that you are at least considering changing your eating habits. Indeed, you may well have tried to do this in the past. As we shall see, change can be difficult, and sometimes we can feel like we are taking one step forward and two steps back. It is really easy to get disheartened and give up, or blame ourselves for our 'weakness'. This chapter will help you understand why 'failure' and setbacks are normal and to be expected as an inevitable part of the process of change. We will explore how to make the most of these setbacks and beat overeating for good.

This chapter is all about preparing you to make changes. By the time you have worked through it you will have the tools to keep you motivated and to understand how and why setbacks take place and respond to them compassionately.

## The seven stages of change

Psychologists have been very interested in how people change. The good news is that people can and do change, and we have much better ideas about how to make this happen than we used to. Two pioneers in this field, James Prochaska and Carlo DiClemente, were particularly interested in helping people give up physically and psychologically addictive behaviour such as smoking and alcohol misuse, and they worked out a model of how change happens that has now been widely applied to a range of difficulties, including eating problems. Many people I have worked with have found this useful in helping them understand where they are in relation to the stages of change and to work out how to move towards permanently beating overeating.

Prochaska and DiClemente identified seven stages in the change process from not thinking about change to changing for good. Let's take a look at how these stages may apply to beating overeating.

## Pre-contemplation

In this stage, we are not trying to address our overeating. We are likely to be caught up in a comfort eating or dieting mindset. We may become quite defensive or dismissive if people talk to us about our overeating, or express concern, or try to stop us comfort eating or dieting.

## Contemplation

Here we are likely to be thinking about or discussing our overeating. For example, you may have been in this stage when you were reading the early chapters of this book. This stage can often be quite distressing, as we think about the impact that overeating has had on us and the various reasons we have needed overeating to help us cope with our situation or emotions. This is a stage that can often be difficult to tolerate, and people often move back into pre-contemplation to avoid this distress. If we are going to beat overeating (or any other problem in our lives, for that matter) it is really important to remember that this suffering is a purposeful step on the journey to change, and not to beat ourselves up for having needed to overeat in the past.

## Preparation

This is a stage in which we are planning to make change and getting ready to move forward. The more time we put into this stage, the better chance we may have of success in making the changes we need to beat overeating. Sometimes we can feel in a rush to do something about our difficulties: this is understandable, but can lead to unintended consequences of change that can accidentally sabotage things later on. The work you have done in completing your personal history, eating diaries and compassionate formulation is part of this stage.

Your compassionate formulation should help you manage some of the unintended consequences of change, but it is important to remember that there is no such thing as 'perfect preparation'. This stage can sometimes feel rather overwhelming, as we notice the many things that overeating may have helped us with. So as part of preparing for change, and the distress it may bring with it for a time, we need to prepare for making small and achievable changes, and to be aware that sometimes change will have unintended consequences, or help us to learn something new about ourselves that will need to be incorporated in our revised formulation and action plans.

## Action

In this stage – covered in the following three chapters of this book – we are putting our plans into action. This is often hard work and can be quite frustrating, but it can also be very satisfying and empowering to learn to new ways to manage life's challenges. Change can be quite a slow process, and there can be unintended consequences or obstacles that we have not planned for. To have the best chance of coping with these, which may seem disheartening at the time, it is really important to have reasons for making this change that are important to you, and ideally also to have support from others. This does not mean that we can't change if we don't have external support. For example, developing a compassionate relationship with yourself and having a strong compassionate image can give you someone in your corner cheering you on and commiserating when things get tough.

## Maintenance

In this stage we tend to find that the changes we have made have become easier to manage. However, sometimes this can lull us into thinking that our old coping styles are changed for good. It can be relatively easy to forget the things that are helping us to beat overeating and to see any setback as a sign that the work we did before was wasted, or anything going wrong as a sign that we are weak in some way.

## Lapse

It's almost inevitable, when we are trying to change previously successful coping strategies and to develop new ways of managing our emotions or overcome old habits, that we will have a lapse or setback at some point. Lapses are more likely to be triggered when our new coping strategies are becoming established. However, they can also occur when we face new or unfamiliar situations. For example, we may have managed to reduce our overeating at home very well, but then go on holiday with friends who encourage us to overeat. Lapses can also occur when we try to push changes too fast – for example, moving quickly from establishing a structured approach to managing our eating to learning to rely on our hunger to inform us when we are full. They key thing here is to have a plan for managing lapses, which sees them as part of a normal learning curve rather than as taking you back to square one.

It is likely that we will sometimes move from a lapse back into a period of pre-contemplation, or even into a prolonged period of overeating. Don't worry: we all go through these times when we are making changes. The key is to learn from our lapses and, when we are ready, to move on to the next phase of the process of change. With practice this process of recovery becomes quicker each time, and indeed you may even learn to welcome the occasional lapse to remind you that you do have the skill and courage to overcome setbacks. Many people find that they feel better about them-selves for knowing that they have the strength to do this.

## Termination

At this point we find that our new strategies have stood the test of time. We have learned to manage and overcome the obstacles to changing our eating habits.

# Why think about the process of change?

The key reasons for thinking about this process are:

- to remind us that we are only human, that change takes time, and that we will all have setbacks;

- to help us recognize what stage we are in and to work with rather than against it: for example, it is OK to think about changing (contemplation) for some time before action, but we may need to plan to support ourselves through any distress this may cause us;

- to help us develop realistic expectations of the amount of time and energy we may need to devote to making changes;

- to develop a sense that facing obstacles and making mistakes is normal and OK.

If we are in the *contemplation* stage, we may need to spend more time thinking about the potential benefits of change, as well as the costs, before we are ready to move on.

If we are in the *preparation* stage, we may need to think about our plans for beating overeating: how we can develop small and achievable targets that will help us towards our goals; any potential obstacles that we're aware of at this stage; the support we might need and where we might get it from; and the skills we may need to develop to help us put our plans into action.

If we are in the *action* phase we may need to think about the amount of time and energy we can devote to changing, how we will keep ourselves motivated and how we will manage lapses.

In the *maintenance* phase we may need to work on recognizing the changes we have made and encouraging ourselves to maintain them, reminding ourselves of the benefits of change, and again to think about how we manage lapses.

## Compassionate motivation

As you may recall from Chapter 4, one of the key attributes of a compassionate mind is compassionate motivation. This comes from a deep caring for the well-being of ourselves and others that generates a decision and commitment to help care for and relieve suffering. As we have seen, sometimes other mindsets can block us from alleviating our suffering, or divert us to short-term solutions to our distress that can inadvertently lead to further suffering in the long run. Compassionate motivation tends to take a longer-term view of caring for ourselves and others, and is also interested in helping us manage the unintended consequences of the ways we manage distress (such as overeating) and in caring for us as we make these longer-term changes.

When we bring this type of motivation together with an understanding of the process of change, the combination can be very powerful in helping us remain motivated in our quest to overcome overeating and in finding ways to give us the best chance of succeeding. It can also help us to understand and deal compassionately with the inevitable lapses and setbacks that occur for everyone who changes their relationship with food.

The exercises below are designed to help you explore and develop your motivation to change. However, before you begin to work though them, it is really important to bring your compassionate mind into play. What we are mainly interested in here is helping you to develop your sense of caring for yourself and your desire to reduce any difficult emotions you may be feeling, particularly in the long term.

So, before you begin each of the exercises below, set aside some time to bring your compassionate image into mind – either your compassionate self or your compassionate companion. Begin by establishing your soothing breathing rhythm. When you are ready, imagine yourself as a deeply compassionate person who fully understands why we overeat, for reasons beyond our control, and why managing eating is hard.

Focus on a sense of warmth and kindness. Let your face settle into a compassionate expression. Imagine how you might speak to someone with gentle understanding and encouragement, and consider what your compassionate tone of voice might sound like.

If you prefer, you can imagine how your compassionate image/companion would motivate you to resolve overeating. In that case you would imagine their dedication to you, their wisdom, kindness and strength. Pay attention to really trying to imagine their compassionate tone of voice.

When you think you have created this mindset, at least to some extent, then you can begin the exercises. Try to spend a couple of minutes on each of the following exercises at first and write down whatever comes to mind. You can return to the exercises whenever you find any new things that might motivate you, or if you find that you lose motivation to work on your overeating.

### EXERCISE 10.1:  WHAT STAGE OF CHANGE AM I IN AND HOW CAN I MOVE FORWARD?

This first exercise helps you to think about what stage of change you are in at the moment. You can then use your compassionate image to help you consider what would help you move into the next phase. Imagine considering and answering this question with kindness, openness, honesty and understanding.

The next exercise is designed to help you if you find that you are in the contemplation and preparation stages of change. It will help you to identify reasons for changing your overeating as well as the benefits of keeping overeating as part of your life.

### EXERCISE 10.2:  RECOGNIZING THE BENEFITS AND COSTS OF OVEREATING

Using all of the information you have gained from your personal history, eating diaries and any other sources, try to complete statements 1–5 below. Your personal compassionate formulation for overeating really comes into its own in helping you to explore your reasons for change here. Remember, your compassionate mind knows that overeating may have been your best coping strategy in the past, and is not going to criticize you for it, only help you to take responsibility for seeking better coping strategies in the future. Keep your compassionate mind uppermost as you then answer questions 6 and 7 with kindness, openness, honesty and understanding.

(1)  My overeating helps me to manage:


(2)  My overeating has had the following unintended consequences on my health:

(3) My overeating has had the following unintended consequences on my mood, thoughts and feelings:

(4) My overeating has had the following unintended consequences on my social life and relationships:

(5) My overeating has had the following unintended consequences on my occupational or academic life:

(6) In what ways would my life improve if I changed my eating habits?

(7) What would motivate me to give up overeating?

When you can answer the last two questions from a compassionate perspective, you are on the way from the contemplation to the preparation stage.

It can be useful to keep your answers to these questions – we can call them your 'motivational lists' – somewhere to provide a daily reminder of why you want to change. People I have worked with have found various ways to do this. They include:

- keeping your motivational lists where you can easily see them (such as on the fridge door or the bathroom mirror, or even as a screen saver!);

- keeping them in a 'beating overeating' scrapbook to which you can add pictures, poems, or letters that can motivate you to change;

- sharing your reasons for changing with someone who cares about you, and giving that person (or people) permission to remind you of why you want to change;

- spending some time each day thinking about the reasons to change from the perspective of your compassionate image.

Please remember that the things that will motivate you are personal to *you*. They may not always make logical sense, and they certainly won't be exactly the same for everyone picking up this book! Different things will motivate you at different times, and again this is perfectly normal. The only real rule that we have about motivation is that it must be compassionate. It must have our best interests at heart and should not involve bullying, cajoling or scaring us into change. This type of behaviour can work in the short term, but further down the line is only likely to result in us being more self-critical and miserable, or even rebelling against the very changes we want to encourage ourselves to make.

## Improving your chances of success: planning for blocks to change

The final element of the preparation stage is to plan for potential blocks to change. Some of these blocks will be specific to the activities and exercises we will use to help us beat overeating, and we will explore these as we introduce each activity. However, there may be more general blocks that we can address before you decide to begin changing your relationship with food and eating.

To resolve overeating you will need to make time for yourself to work on the exercises in the book. On average this will take about an hour a day – usually in short bursts (for example, spending a minute of so after each eating episode recording the details in your diary). However, sometimes you may need to set aside an hour to plan your eating, or write a compassionate letter (which we will look at in Chapter 14). Finding this time can be very difficult, even if we really want to, so it is important that you see the work from the perspective of caring for yourself, and truly wanting to alleviate your suffering, rather than as something you have to criticize or bully yourself into doing!

Sometimes the commitments we have in our lives, or the people around us, can make it difficult to make the changes we want to. Again, it can be helpful to think about this in advance, especially if we can break this obstacle down into practical difficulties that we could find ways of working around to give us the best chance of making permanent changes in ways we eat.

You can use the next two exercises to think about any practical difficulties before we move towards developing the first phase of your action plan for beating overeating – planning to eat differently. Again, your compassionate image's perspective will be helpful here; it knows the difference between your fears of change and the real obstacles that we can all face in dealing with our problems in the longer term. It is wise enough to help you manage some of these practical problems without blaming you, or being angry with you, for the things that may slow you down as you overcome overeating. Imagine doing this with kindness, openness, honesty and understanding.

### EXERCISE 10.3: IDENTIFYING PRACTICAL PROBLEMS

Make a note of any practical problems that your compassionate image can see that may make it difficult for you to make time to change your overeating. For example, you may be just starting a new job, or moving house, and this may leave you very little time to do your compassion exercises or to plan your eating.

### EXERCISE 10.4: OVERCOMING PRACTICAL PROBLEMS

Now use your compassionate image to help you plan how you might overcome some of these practical difficulties. So, you may decide to postpone starting your journey to eating compassionately until the house move is complete, or you have settled into the new job. Or, knowing that the events coming up are going to be stressful, you may decide to take some time out to do your exercises and to eat regularly. Both are examples of a compassionate solution if they recognize your limitations and support you to work with them, without criticizing yourself for the solution you have chosen.

## Some things to try

While I can't know, of course, what your personal obstacles are, it might be helpful for you to consider how people have managed to overcome some of the common obstacles you may well encounter.

### Making time to plan

In the early stages of this process you may need to learn to make time and space to eat and to reflect on your feelings. Start to make this time before you start to change your eating; for example, plan a few more breaks in the day; don't rush straight to the next thing after you finish the meals you already have; try to create five minutes of 'me time' every couple of hours.

### Focus your attention on changing

This can be difficult, too. There are so many other things that can pull us away, and it is very easy to fall back into old habits. Try to set up reminders of the times that you are going to eat (perhaps as an alarm call on your phone).

### Maintaining attention on the reasons and triggers for overeating

For example, you might put a note on you fridge that says, 'Do I really want to eat now?' Perhaps you can keep a notebook or send yourself a text message for when you spot an urge to overeat, or when you have found a new way to cope.

### Staying focused on why you are doing the work

Many people – perhaps most – get disheartened when they're trying to change things, and it will be relatively easy to go back to not working on overeating, especially at first. Keep the motivational lists that you made in Exercise 10.2 somewhere you can look at them; maybe even do them again when you notice that you want to give up, or have had a lapse.

Another way to stay focused is to keep a scrapbook of the reasons why you want to change; this can include pictures, drawing, poetry, artwork – anything you like, really. The key is to make it personal to the reasons you want to change and to the kind of person you want to become.

## Focus on success

People who overeat are often quite self-critical and tend to focus on their mistakes. It can help to get into the habit of writing down every day each small (or big) step you have taken in improving your eating and becoming more compassionate. You might want to keep this list in your scrapbook and look at it each morning when you get up!

Sometimes what we initially think are practical blocks (e.g. 'I don't have time') turn out to be linked to emotional blocks (e.g. 'I am worried what people will think of me if I make more time for myself') or to other worries about changing (e.g. 'How will I deal with my feelings if I can't use food when I am upset?'). It is absolutely normal to have both practical and emotional blocks to change. They key thing is to be compassionate about our limitations and with our concerns about changing.

It is helpful to be aware that the more blocks there are to our progress the longer it may take us to beat overeating – but that does not mean we can't do it. The biggest single factor in predicting whether we will succeed is our desire for and commitment to change. This is why it's important to work out why you want to change your overeating and what will help keep you motivated when the going gets tough.

## Getting support to help you resolve overeating

Overeating is something that many people feel ashamed of, and this can stop them from seeking appropriate support. This is something else that can undermine our chances of beating overeating, or at least lengthen the time it takes. The next exercise involves using your compassionate image to help you make a list all of the people who might support you. Again, your image will be wise enough to know the difference between the fears that may stop you asking them to help, and the reality of whether these people would genuinely want to help and support you.

Your list could include family, friends, work colleagues, your doctor and perhaps a therapist. Of course, you may not wish to share everything about yourself with everyone on your list – in fact, some people can help without ever knowing you have a problem. For example, you may arrange to go out with someone because you enjoy their company, and when you are with them you are less likely to overeat. There may be other people in your life who care for you and perhaps have a more compassionate view of you than you have of yourself. People like this can be really helpful in steering us away from the urge to beat ourselves up for overeating, or drawing our attention to aspects of ourselves that our self-critical or dieting mindsets do not.

As with all the exercises, consider the task with kindness, openness, honesty and understanding.

### EXERCISE 10.5: IDENTIFYING SOURCES OF HELP

Use your compassionate image to help you list the people who could help you beat overeating and what kind of help they may be able to give you (e.g. practical, emotional, distraction etc).

*Person*                    *Kind of help*

When you have developed your own plan for beating overeating, you may wish to talk with some of these people about how they can help. You may also wish to share this book with them and let them see your compassionate formulation, or other elements of your action plan to beat overeating.

## Compassionately managing setbacks

As we saw earlier, setbacks are to be expected when we try to change the way we eat (or anything else, for that matter). Again, we need to bring our compassionate mind to bear when we have a setback or lapse into overeating. If you were truly motivated to care for yourself, and to learn from and move forward from a setback, what kind of things would your compassionate self say? Would it blame you, see you as inadequate or weak in some way? Or would it want to comfort and support you, to help you understand and learn from your setbacks?

Of course, in the disappointment of having experienced a setback it may not be easy to maintain your compassionate mindset. So it's a good idea to practise in advance how you might respond when it happens. To do this, first bring your compassionate mind into play. Now imagine that you are supporting a friend who has tried to change their overeating but has had a setback – perhaps has lapsed back into overeating because they had gone to a party, or found out some upsetting news. How would you feel if you wanted them to do well but had seen them struggle? What sort of thing would you like to say to them to help them be compassionately motivated to learn from the experience and to make a renewed commitment to continuing to work on their overeating?

When you have some idea of the things that your compassionate self would like to say to someone else, you could try writing a short compassionate letter to yourself that you can keep to read when lapses occur. (We'll look at writing compassionate letters in detail in Chapter 14.) This might include expressing your appreciation of your courage and wisdom for working on overeating, your sadness and your disappointment for the lapse, but also your support and encouragement for continuing the journey. You may also want to put down some ideas for the things that can help remotivate you and the names of people who could support you.

**SUMMARY**

In this chapter we have explored the process of change and, using your compassionate mind, helped you to develop an understanding of your current stage of motivation and to identify ways of supporting yourself as you move forward. We have also explored how to deal compassionately with the lapses that are inevitable as you change your eating habits, and how to treat them as important new learning opportunities, rather than seeing them as failures or insurmountable obstacles.

In the next chapter we will work on the first stage of a compassionate action plan to address the practical elements of changing our eating patterns: finding out the amount and types of foods we eat, and how to provide our body with the physical activity and rest it needs to keep us healthy.

# 11 Working out what your body needs

In the previous chapter we explored how to develop your motivation for working on overeating. By now I hope you are clearer about the reasons why you overeat and the intended and unintended consequences of overeating, the reasons why you want to change your eating habits, and some of the blocks that may get in the way. As the next step forward, this chapter focuses on our physical needs for food, activity and rest. It will show you how to work out your own personal energy needs, so that in the chapters that follow you can use this information in working out a new approach to eating.

Caring for ourselves and others involves, among other things, a concern for our and their physical and emotional well-being. Therefore a compassionate action plan to address overeating needs to address both of these areas of our lives in aiming to develop a new relationship with our eating and our body. This will include aiming to stop using food to manage our emotions.

Caring about our physical well-being includes:

- eating as much as our body needs;

- balancing our energy intake through the day;

- providing our body with the nutrients that it needs;

- providing our body with foods that will help us to feel full and satisfied;

- providing our body with enough physical activity to keep it healthy;

- providing our body with adequate time to rest and repair itself.

Caring about our emotional needs includes:

- managing our emotional regulation systems (the 'three circles');

- developing a range of coping strategies to deal with various kinds of threat;

- developing emotional resilience to manage life's challenges and setbacks;

- allowing ourselves to experience joy and pleasure, including enjoying eating.

## Looking after our physical needs

As we have seen, our comfort food, dieting and other eating mindsets can lead us to eat in ways that do not meet our physical needs. To recap, unless we eat enough satisfying food on a regular basis, we are very likely to overeat (as well as to experience a whole range of physical and psychological problems), but if we regularly eat more than we need we are likely to weigh more than we should and be at more risk of certain health problems. Therefore the ways we eat, and the amount and types of food we eat, can be critical in addressing overeating.

We are a species that evolved to be physically active – indeed, physical activity can have the same effect as anti-depressant medication in improving our mood. Yet in the West many of us have become very sedentary. If we are aiming to develop a compassionate mind approach to our body we may also need to think about our relationship with physical activity. We need about an hour of physical activity a day that raises our heart rate but leaves us able to hold a conversation while we are doing it. However, it is important to take medical advice before you start taking more exercise, particularly if you have been inactive for a while.

Many of us lead very busy lives that do not take account of our body's needs to rest and repair. Indeed, lack of sleep has been associated with mood problems and a tendency to overeat. Again, we will need to take this into account as we develop a compassionate relationship with our body. It's recommended that most adults have seven or eight hours' sleep a night.

Many of you reading this book will be looking to it to help you lose weight. That is absolutely OK *as long as you are actually overweight*. As we have seen, being overweight can pose physical health problems, although perhaps not as many as we are often led to believe. A compassionate mind approach to our body may result in our losing weight if overeating leads us consistently to eat more than our body needs, or if we have experienced the yo-yo weight loss and gain that is usually associated with dieting. However, that is not the main aim of taking a more compassionate approach to your body's needs. *The main aim is to learn to feed your body and provide it with appropriate activity to keep it as healthy as possible, and to help you to find and live with the body that your genetic history meant you to live in.* This can be a difficult journey as our emotions and eating habits can become very entangled, so it is also likely we will need to address our emotional needs along the way.

## What does your body need?

Working out *exactly* what any individual's body needs is quite a complex activity, taking into account their body's energy requirements by the hour, their exact weight, their gender, metabolic rate and a whole range of other variables. This can be done, and indeed the guidelines we are going to work from now are based on these types of calculations. But of course, the level of expertise and time required to do this individually is unlikely to be available to most of us. The good news is that there is relatively little difference in our energy needs, leaving aside those of us who have severe medical conditions or who are elite athletes. This means that it is OK for the rest of us to work from the general guidance about our nutritional needs – which says, as we have already seen, that most women need about 2,000 calories a day, and most men about 2,500 calories a day.

But the number of calories that we eat is only part of the story. Our body also needs a range of foods to keep us healthy. Nutritional guidelines place these foods into five categories and suggest the approximate balance between these categories that will help keep us healthy. These groups are:

- starchy foods (carbohydrates);

- fruit and vegetables;

- meat, fish, eggs and beans (proteins);

- milk and dairy foods (or substitutes such as soya milk);

- foods containing fat and sugar.

*Starchy foods* include bread, cereals, potatoes, pasta, maize and cornbread; there is also starch in beans, lentils, peas, breadfruit and cassava. All these foods contain carbohydrates, which are an essential source of energy. In a healthy diet, starchy foods should make up around a third of everything we eat.

*Fruit and vegetables* are a vital source of vitamins and minerals, and nutritional guidelines suggest we eat five portions of them a day. One apple, banana, pear or similar-sized fruit is one portion. A slice of pineapple or melon is one portion and three heaped tablespoons of vegetables is another. A glass of fruit juice also counts as one portion. Juice only counts as one of your five a day, no matter how much you drink.

*Meat, fish, eggs and beans* are all sources of protein, which is essential for the growth and repair of the body. Around 15 per cent of the calories we eat each day should come from protein. Meat is a good source of protein, as well as of many vitamins and minerals. Fish is another important source of protein. There is evidence that people who eat two portions or more a week of oily fish (such as sardines, mackerel, herring and salmon) are at lower risk of heart disease. That's because oily fish contains high levels of a 'good fat' called omega-3. Eggs, pulses (e.g. beans and lentils), nuts and seeds are also great sources of protein.

*Milk and dairy foods* such as cheese and yoghurt are other good sources of protein. They also contain calcium, which helps keep bones healthy.

*Fats and sugar* are powerful sources of energy for the body. Fat has been divided into two groups:

- Saturated fats are concentrated in such foods as pies, meat products, sausages, cakes and biscuits: these can raise your cholesterol level and increase your risk of heart disease. Most of us in the UK eat too much saturated fat, putting us at risk of health problems.

- Unsaturated fats, on the other hand, provide us with the essential fatty acids needed to stay healthy and can actually lower your cholesterol level. Oily fish, nuts and seeds, avocados, olive oil and other vegetable oils are sources of unsaturated fat.

There are two kinds of food containing sugar, too:

- Naturally occurring sugar, in foods such as fruit and milk, tends to be released slowly from food.

- Added sugar appears in processed foods such as fizzy drinks, cakes, biscuits, chocolate, pastries, ice cream and jam. It's also in some ready-made savoury foods such as pasta sauces and baked beans. This added sugar tends to be released more quickly from food and so can lead to rapid swings in blood sugar, which can leave us feeling tired and hungry.

Table 11.1 sets out how the recommended proportions of these different types of food in a healthy diet translate into the calories you need from each

Table 11.1: Approximate daily calorie needs and balance of food types

| Food type and ideal proportion of daily calories | Calories per day (for a woman) | Calories per day (for a man) |
|---|---|---|
| Starch (30%) | 600 | 750 |
| Fruit and vegetables (30%) | 600 | 750 |
| Protein – meat, fish, eggs and beans (15%) | 300 | 375 |
| Milk and dairy (15%) | 300 | 375 |
| Fat and sugar (10%) | 200 | 250 |
| Total (100%) | 2,000 | 2,500 |

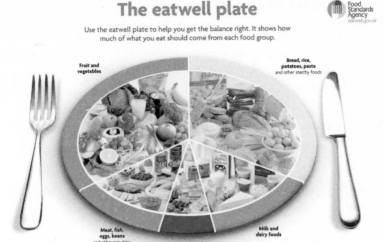

**Figure 11.1:** The 'eatwell plate'

*Source*: http://www.eatwell.gov.uk/healthydiet/eatwellplate
Reproduced with permission.

type every day. These are amounts for the average woman or man; of course, if you are very physically active you will need to add additional calories to meet increased demands on your body.

If you find visual images easier to remember than numbers, you may find the 'eatwell plate' shown in Figure 11.1 helpful. This is another way of showing the same information about the proportions of the various food types we need.

Interestingly, these different food types have different effects on our satiety system. This is the system that makes us feel full and satisfied, so we know when we have eaten enough. Some foods are better than others at doing this. Protein is the most effective food for doing this, followed by starchy foods; both are better at helping us feel full and satisfied than foods whose calorie content consists largely of sugar or fat. In fact, eating sugary foods can lead to a temporary rise in blood sugar, followed by a rapid drop, leaving us hungrier, low in mood, and more tired than before!

To help us overcome overeating it is really important that we eat:

- enough calories for our body's needs;

- regularly, to avoid the blood sugar drops that provoke overeating;

- a varied range of food, with a healthy balance between the types of food we eat.

If we do all three of these things it will help us to learn to recognize and respond to our bodies' sensations of feeling hungry and feeling full.

## Moving towards balanced eating that meets your needs

Ideally, eating compassionately would mean that we understand what our body needs and when it needs it, and allow ourselves to enjoy the foods we like in a way that does not affect our health or lead to overeating. That can feel like a really tall order if we have been struggling with overeating, or denying ourselves food, for any length of time. Sometimes even thinking about this as a goal can lead us to give up, believing that this *may* be possible for some people, but certainly isn't for us!

Well, if you're thinking this, you certainly won't be alone. Remember, our see-food-and-eat-it brain, and the comfort eating, dieting and other eating mindsets we develop, may take us a long way from compassionate eating. So although this may be our goal, it is unlikely that any of us will be able to do this 100 per cent of the time. The good news is that occasionally eating in a less compassionate way (for example, overindulging in the holidays) is something that our body can cope with relatively well; it just can't cope if we do it a lot of the time.

Many people I have worked with have found it very helpful to have a structure to guide them in learning to eat compassionately. This involves putting some time into planning what and when we are going to eat, and then gradually learning to recognize our body's signals for hunger and fullness and to respond to these. Making these changes can provoke a whole range of thoughts and feelings which can stop us from compassionately caring for our body. We will explore ways to work on these in more detail in the next chapter. For now, we will just work on developing your skills in estimating how much you need to eat and how much you eat at the moment.

## Working out what you're eating now

In the early stages of learning to eat compassionately you will need to devote a little time to working out what you are currently eating, and how this compares to what you need. This can be a little unnerving at first, especially if you have been used to calorie counting as part of a dieting mindset or if you are not used to being aware of what you eat. However, if you are going to work out what your body needs, you will need to know how much energy you take in, how much energy you use up, and how the types of food that you eat relate to the types of food your body needs.

If you have worked through the book to this point, you will already have had a go at keeping an eating diary. We can now use this, along with a calorie-counting book or website, to estimate your energy needs and your energy intake. There are many commercial and open access internet sites that give the calorie values of a wide range of foods, as well as a range of calorie-counting books in the shops and libraries. Many also tell you how many calories you use up doing different kinds of activity/exercise. I suggest that you look at a few so you can choose one that you find easy to use.

Like all tools, knowledge about the calories of the food we eat and the energy we use can potentially have some unintended consequences. These include:

- activating our dieting mindset;

- reminding us of negative experiences in the past with calorie counting;

- becoming obsessed with the calories we eat;

- using calorie estimating to beat ourselves up for being greedy, out of control, etc.

So, before we begin it is really important that you explore and manage these possibilities from the perspective of your compassionate mind. Take a little time to engage your soothing system by using your soothing breathing rhythm; then, when you are ready, bring your compassionate image to mind. Allow yourself to experience its care and warmth for you and then gently try to 'step into' its shoes. Let yourself imagine that you truly want to care for yourself, to offer yourself the benefits of it strength, courage and wisdom in exploring the next two exercises.

### EXERCISE 11.1: IDENTIFYING DIFFICULTIES IN CALORIE ESTIMATING

Allow your compassionate image to identify any difficulties it can foresee if you were to work out the calories you have eaten, and jot them down in the space below.

- 
- 
- 
- 

Once you are aware of these risks, you can then use your compassionate image to help you to develop a plan to manage them. Please remember that the aim of estimating calories here is to help you to understand and to care for your body's needs; it is not about losing weight or beating yourself up for overeating. If you notice your critical mindset chipping in, it is really important to slow down and return to your compassionate image before you go on with the task. You may wish to do this in the form of a compassionate letter (see Chapter 14 for more on how to do this), or just to jot the main points down in the space below in Exercise 11.2.

### EXERCISE 11.2: MY COMPASSIONATE THOUGHTS AND ACTIONS FOR MANAGING ESTIMATING MY ENERGY INTAKE

- 
- 
- 
-

The benefits of spending a short period of your life becoming more aware of what you eat and learning to eat in a way that cares for your body's needs can be really worth the time and effort it takes. People I have worked with have told me that this knowledge gives them control over what and how they want to eat, and makes it far easier to manage their biological urges that used to cause them to overeat. The good news is that you will only need to estimate your calories in a lot of detail once during the whole programme, when you are working out your first meal plan. You can use the information you have gathered from your diaries so far to do this. Ideally, use at least two weeks' worth of diaries, particularly if there are big variations in how much you eat or how much activity you do.

It is a lot easier to estimate your energy balance when you have a meal plan in place, as you can simply add or subtract calorie estimates for food you eat in addition to the plan, or for foods you leave out, as well as increases or decreases in your activity levels.

You can use the following guidelines to help you with this task:

- Estimate calories. You don't need to weigh out to the ounce everything that you eat – a good estimate is usually good enough.

- Note all the physical activities you do in fifteen-minute episodes.

- Make a note of the types of food that you eat, and approximately how many calories per day of each of the five main food types you eat.

Let's think about what this would look like in practice by exploring Alison's diary again. To save you flicking back to Chapter 8, the same day's diary is reproduced again here as Figure 11.2. Alison was not particularly active on this Monday, so her energy requirement would have been the normal 2,000 calories. However, if Alison was more active, as she was on the Tuesday, we would need to raise her energy need to take this into account. For example, on Tuesday she spent four hours doing housework, and two hours doing exercise. We used a calorie-counting book to work out her energy needs for three hours of housework (720 calories) and two hours doing exercise (two aerobic classes at the gym: 840 calories). We did not include one hour of the housework, as this would have been included

| Monday 23 March | | Overeating? Yes/No | Dieting mindset or comfort food mindset active when eating? Yes/No | Thoughts and feelings |
|---|---|---|---|---|
| Situation Where were you? Who were you with? How were you feeling? What were you thinking before you ate? | What you ate or drank (type and amount) Physical activity (type and duration) | | | These can be thoughts and feelings during or after eating, about doing the diary, or anything else that you think is important |
| 8 a.m., at home, alone A bit hungry, tired Not really thinking about anything | Cereal, 2 slices of toast, tea | No | No | Felt OK about eating, a bit worried about going to work today |
| 10 a.m., at work, with colleagues A bit anxious Worried about difficult meeting later today | Tea and 5 ginger biscuits | Yes | Comfort food | Felt a little worried that colleagues would think I was greedy, but felt I needed the food to calm me down |
| 12.30 p.m., at work, alone A bit queasy, not hungry More anxious about meeting | Tea and 10 more biscuits Had planned to have lunch but couldn't face it | Maybe? | Comfort, but also thought I would cut back on the biscuits for the rest of the week | Felt greedy |

| | | | | |
|---|---|---|---|---|
| 1.45 p.m. at restaurant, alone. Very upset by meeting, felt angry with boss and useless. Mainly thinking about meeting and worried about what other people thought about me | Burger meal, large milkshake | No | Mainly comfort but planned not to eat for the rest of the day | Felt OK about eating, but very down about myself, worried about going back to work |
| 10.30 p.m. home, with partner. Still upset about work. Felt I deserved a treat | 4 glasses of wine, takeaway meal, plus leftovers. Individual tub of ice cream | Yes | Dieting mind until just before the meal, but partner came in from work late and brought in a takeaway | Didn't want to eat, but when I did felt out of control and could not stop. Felt angry with myself for overeating, planning to eat a lot less tomorrow |

**Figure 11.2:** Alison's eating diary

in Alison's routine energy needs. So on Tuesday Alison needed around 3,560 calories to meet her energy needs.

You can see from this that physical activity can make a big difference to how much we need to eat. It is really important to take this into account when we are trying to understand daily fluctuations in our energy needs, and how hungry we are likely to be!

If we go back to Alison's eating diary for Monday, we can add up approximately how many calories she ate and drank:

1 bowl of cereal with skimmed milk and sugar = 200 calories

2 slices of toast and butter = 300 calories

15 ginger biscuits = 750 calories

Burger meal (small cheeseburger, no chips), large milkshake = 700 calories

4 (small) glasses of red wine = 350 calories

Takeaway meal (pizza, 4 slices) = 1,280 calories

Individual tub of ice cream = 180 calories

3 cups of tea with skimmed milk = 30 calories

*Total calories = 3,790*

This would have been only a little more than she needed on Tuesday, but was 1,790 calories more than the 2,000 her body needed on Monday. One of the typical patterns that we can fall into when we overeat is to try to make up for it the next day (hence Alison's very active day on Tuesday after she had overeaten on Monday). Although Alison's energy intake across the two days more or less balances out, the problem was that she swung between overeating one day and then not eating enough for her needs the next day. By the time she reached Wednesday she was back to overeating because she became very hungry after leaving herself so short of the energy she needed on Tuesday. We will explore how to address this issue when we come to meal planning in the next chapter.

The other interesting thing that Alison discovered from her diary was that most of her calories came from foods high in fat and sugar, such as biscuits, or high in carbohydrate, like cereal, bread and pizza. She also tended to have quite a lot of dairy products, such as milk and milkshakes, and a significant percentage of her calories came from alcohol. Her protein intake was relatively small (mainly the meat in her burger), and she had no fruit or vegetables on Monday. The difficulty here was that the high-energy foods she ate were also the foods that she found least filling, and so she tended to eat more of them.

Ideally, Alison needed to significantly increase her intake of foods that were less high in energy but would help fill her up (such as fruit and vegetables). She also needed to swap her high-energy foods for others that included more protein, which again would be more filling than fatty and sugary foods such as biscuits. This was bound to be difficult, as sweet and fatty foods can directly soothe us and so tend to be the comfort foods of choice for most of us. Still, with time and perseverance Alison was able to make significant changes in her energy intake and to change the balance of the food types she ate.

Alison also learned to develop other ways to cope with the low moods and distress that she had got used to relieving by eating. She learned to lower her 'emotional temperature' by introducing a number of self-soothing activities into her daily routine – such as ensuring she had at least a thirty-minute 'me time' bath every evening. She also practised using her safe place imagery to help her regain some emotional stability when she got upset – in fact she got so good at this that she was able to summon up a feeling of being soothed by just imagining a peaceful beach for a couple of seconds! Alison also built a number of distractions into her routine, even including her partner in a salsa dance class.

Like many of us, Alison tended to estimate the calories she had eaten in relation to how she felt about food. For example, she believed her biscuits, which were high in fat and sugar, contained far fewer calories than her breakfast, as breakfast tended to be more filling. She was feeling quite upset when she had her burger, and greedy when she had her takeaway, so she tended to overestimate what she had eaten on these occasions. She often associated feeling full with feeling greedy or having overeaten. She found it really helpful to work out realistic calorie estimates for these eating episodes and to see how they differed from her 'feeling-based' calorie estimates.

## Working out your energy balance

Our energy balance is the difference between the amount of energy we take in and the amount of energy we need to fuel our bodily systems and whatever else we do. Most people who overeat will have a positive energy balance (they eat more than they need), but on some days they may have a negative energy balance (eating less than they need). A long-term positive energy balance leads to weight gain, while severe short- and medium-term negative energy balances tend to lead to overeating. In this section we are interested in helping you develop a more neutral energy balance to help reduce overeating that is based on feeling hungry. This will also help to stabilize your weight so that you do not need to get into a dieting mindset to manage it.

As we have already seen, there are two elements to our daily energy needs: our basic energy needs (2,000 calories for a woman, 2,500 for a man) and the energy we use up above our normal energy needs (for example, through housework, walking, or formal exercise such as playing football or going to the gym).

It's best to work out our energy balance over a week, as it can fluctuate quite a lot from one day to the next. The easiest way of doing this is to calculate energy intake and energy used for each day and then add them up at the end of the week. You can record these details in Worksheet 10. (There are a couple more blank copies at the back of the book that you can photocopy if you wish.)

As well as the amount of food we eat, we are also interested in eating more of the foods that can keep us healthy and feeling satisfied. So Worksheet 10 also gives you space to record what you are eating and the food type it belongs to. You can then work out the approximate proportion of each type of food you eat in your total intake.

Worksheet 10a: Daily food intake and energy balance

(a) Daily record

| Food eaten | Approximate energy intake (calories) | Main food type (starch, fruit/veg., protein, dairy, sugar/fat) | Activity and approximate energy used |
|---|---|---|---|
| | | | |
| | | | |

**Worksheet 10b: Daily food intake and energy balance**

(b) Daily and weekly summary

| | Monday | Tuesday | Wednesday | Thursday | Friday | Saturday | Sunday | Weekly summary |
|---|---|---|---|---|---|---|---|---|
| Total calorie intake | | | | | | | | |
| Starch | | | | | | | | |
| Fruit and vegetables | | | | | | | | |
| Protein | | | | | | | | |
| Dairy | | | | | | | | |
| Sugar and fat | | | | | | | | |
| Alcohol | | | | | | | | |
| Energy need (=2,000 for female/ 2,500 for male + extra for energy expended in activity) | | | | | | | | |
| Energy balance (= calorie intake − energy need) | | | | | | | | |

We are also interested in the amount of activity we undertake, as the other half of our energy balance equation is how much energy we use up. We can then work out whether we are eating more or less than we need each day, and across the week.

When you have all this information you will be able to use it as the basis for the next stage in changing your eating habits, which is planning your meals to incorporate changes in the amounts and types of foods you eat. This will be the focus of the next chapter.

Exercise 11.3 will take you through some steps to help you complete the worksheet. You might also like to look at Figure 11.3, which is a sample completed copy of the worksheet based on Alison's eating diary for Monday.

As you can see, the first part of Worksheet 10 has spaces for you to record the food you eat, your approximate energy intake (in calories) from it, the type of food it belongs to, and any physical activity. This includes formal exercise, but also day-to-day things like housework or walking. In the second part of the worksheet you can note down your calorie totals (both consumed and used) to arrive at energy balance figures for each day, and then for the whole week.

We are particularly interested here not only in whether you end up with a positive or negative energy balance, but also in what food types you're mostly eating. You can use the 'eatwell plate' and the information in Table 11.1 to guide you in allocating a food type to what you eat. For example, ginger biscuits do contain a lot of starch, but they are included in the 'Sugar and fat' column for Alison's worksheet because this is where they appear on the 'eatwell plate'.

When you are working out your energy balance you will need to spend a little time reflecting on the types of activity you did each day. Many people are surprised by just how active they are, and this in itself can sometimes account for some apparent 'overeating'. As we saw in Chapter 2, if you are lying in bed doing nothing all day, you will need around 1,600 calories just to 'tick over'. If you do a sedentary job with about an hour's worth of physical activity (say, walking to the office and back and around the shops

**(a) Daily record**

| Food eaten | Approximate energy intake (calories) | Main food type (starch, fruit/veg., protein, dairy, sugar/fat) | Activity and approximate energy used |
|---|---|---|---|
| Cereal | 120 | Starch | 30 minutes walking to work (100 calories) |
| Skimmed milk (breakfast) | 80 | Dairy | 30 minutes housework (100 calories) |
| 2 slices toast | 220 | Starch | |
| Butter | 80 | Dairy | |
| Tea with skimmed milk | 30 | Dairy | 30 minute exercise video (only did 10 minutes – 120 calories) |
| Ginger biscuits | 750 | Fat and sugar | |
| Burger bun Burger | 300 100 | Starch Protein | |
| Milk shake | 300 | Dairy | |
| Pizza | 1,280 | Starch | |
| Ice cream | 180 | Dairy | |
| Wine | 350 | Alcohol | |

(b) Daily and weekly summary

| | Monday | Tuesday | Wednesday | Thursday | Friday | Saturday | Sunday | Weekly summary |
|---|---|---|---|---|---|---|---|---|
| Total calorie intake | 3,790 | | | | | | | |
| Starch | 1,920 | | | | | | | |
| Fruit and vegetables | 0 | | | | | | | |
| Protein | 100 | | | | | | | |
| Dairy | 670 | | | | | | | |
| Sugar and fat | 750 | | | | | | | |
| Alcohol | 350 | | | | | | | |
| Energy need (=2000+extra for energy expended in activity) | 2,000 +120 | | | | | | | |
| Energy balance (=calorie intake—energy need) | +1,670 | | | | | | | |

**Figure 11.3:** Alison's daily food intake and energy balance

at lunchtime) you will need 2,000 calories if you are an adult woman and 2,500 calories if you are an adult man. So if you are more active than this you will need to increase your energy intake accordingly – keeping roughly to the same proportions of food types as set out in Table 11.1. For example, if you do an extra hour in the gym you may need an extra 300 calories during the course of the day, ideally in the form of 90 calories of starch, 90 calories of fruit and vegetables, 45 calories of meat, fish eggs, or beans, 45 calories of dairy products and 30 calories of fat and sugar. You will also need some extra fluid to replace what you will lose though perspiration – and a bit of rest to let your body recover!

When you are familiar with the worksheet, and have looked though Alison's example in Figure 11.3, you are ready to think about doing Exercise 11.3.

The key to this exercise is to use your compassionate mind to explore your food diary and complete Worksheet 10 with an approach of gentle curiosity:

- *Gentleness* is important because this exercise can lead us to feeling disappointed, angry or ashamed of what and how we eat, so we really do need to be kind to ourselves and compassionate with the struggles we have with eating. Your compassionate mind can use your personal formulation to help you understand why you eat the way you do and to support and value your commitment to changing the way you eat.

- *Curiosity* is also important, because exploring the types and amounts of food we eat can often provide us with new insights into and understanding of our relationship with food and the areas we feel we can begin to work on. Many people I have worked with have found that taking a kindly, enquiring perspective can help them overcome their usual pattern of either avoiding thinking about what they eat or attacking themselves for what and how they eat.

Remember, you only need to work out your energy balance and the types of food you have eaten in detail once in the whole process of beating overeating, to give you an idea of your current eating pattern and to help you to work out your first meal plan. Doing it in this degree of detail for any longer will become a chore at the very least, and at worst can be counter-productive, as constantly counting the calories of everything you eat is likely to activate your dieting mindset. Once you've done this one-off exercise it is far more helpful to begin to plan your eating in advance, and then review it at the end of the week to see if there are times when you have varied from your plan; then you can refine it, or address things that have led to overeating, as part of the plan for the following week.

Only begin Exercise 11.3 when you feel emotionally ready and practically prepared to start to make changes in your overeating. It is designed to help to you make sense of some of the changes you may need to make. You may need to do a little preparation before you begin. The exercise can take about two hours in total, so you need to set aside time when you can work on it, either all in one go or in several shorter sessions. It can also activate difficult thoughts and feelings and memories in us, particularly if we have dieted a lot in the past or are critical of our eating. So we will need our compassionate mind to guide us, support us through the process, and help us to tolerate any distress that the activity may cause us. Your compassionate mind will be wise enough to know how much of this you can manage at any one time. It can also be helpful to have some self-soothing or other distress management activities pre-arranged for when you finish the exercise.

### EXERCISE 11.3: WORKING OUT YOUR OWN ENERGY BALANCE

Begin by using your safe place image or soothing breathing rhythm to bring your soothing system into play. It is common for people doing this exercise to find that their mind wanders even more frequently than usual; this may be because they have associated looking at what they eat with the urge to diet or self-criticism. If it does, remember to use our motto of 'notice and return' to gently refocus your attention on the task in hand.

When you can feel that your soothing system is uppermost, you are ready to move on to the next stage of the exercise – activating your compassionate image. Allow yourself to experience its compassion for your courage and wisdom in taking on the task of exploring your diary. What sort of things would it say to support you in exploring your diary? How would it encourage you to explore it compassionately rather than using it as a way of motivating you to eat less, or punishing you for eating too much?

You can then, supported by your compassionate image, explore your eating diary from the perspective of your compassionate mind – or, if you find it easier, from the perspective of your compassionate image. This may enable you to explore the diary in a more detached way, almost as if it were someone else's, but still with gentle, compassionate curiosity. Either of these approaches is fine. You may find it easier just to work though one day at a time, and to do the exercise over several days, before you add up your week and summarize the information on Worksheet 10.

However you do this, take your time over it. It is an important part of the groundwork for all the other things you will do to change your relationship with food, eating and your body, so you deserve some time to spend doing it at a pace you can manage.

When you have finished filling in the worksheet, you can explore what your compassionate image would say about what you have learned, and what changes in the amount you eat, the types of food you eat and the activity that you do you could work on. You may wish to jot these thoughts down on paper, perhaps in the form of a compassionate letter (see Chapter 14 for more on how to do this), to guide the efforts to address your overeating that you are now ready to begin.

### SUMMARY

This chapter has explored what being compassionate with our body's needs means, particularly in terms of our need for energy, activity and rest. We have explored a way of using a week's worth of records from your food diary to help you work out your energy balance and the types of food you eat. You can now use this as the basis for developing your plan for changing your eating, and of course working on the thoughts and feelings that lead to overeating, or that may follow from changing your eating. The next two chapters will guide you though a step-by-step approach to doing this compassionately.

# 12 Towards a new way of eating: the first steps

This chapter brings together all the work you have done so far to put together a practical plan for addressing overeating and caring for your body. It shows you how to establish a basic structure for eating that includes managing foods that can put you at risk of overeating. As always, the key is to use your compassionate mind, based on wisdom, kindness and a genuine desire to be encouraging and supportive, to guide you.

## The six-step programme: an outline

In the early stages of building this new relationship with food and your body, you will need to spend time planning when, how and what you are going to eat. The longer you spend doing this – three to six months is probably a good period to aim at – the more likely you are to establish a new eating routine. Then, gradually, you can become less strict with your meal plans, experiment with a wider range of foods, and learn to respond to your experiences of being hungry and full.

Many people confuse meal planning with dieting. Meal planning is not a diet. It is about making changes in our eating pattern, and later in the amounts and types of food we eat. It does this by taking away the option of eating less later if (for any reason) we overeat, as we know we will still stick to eating the next meal we have planned. Meal planning can also help us to change some of the common features of chaotic eating patterns, such as leaving long periods between meals, or eating very frequently, that can put us out of touch with our feelings of hunger and fullness.

Our new way of eating involves learning to be more mindful of the influences that can lead to overeating. It is broken down into six steps:

(1) establishing a regular eating pattern;

(2) reducing our intake of high-risk foods that trigger overeating;

(3) balancing our energy intake with our energy needs;

(4) developing a healthy nutritional balance;

(5) learning to respond to our hunger and fullness;

(6) learning to enjoy food and eating.

Each step will help you learn more about your relationship with overeating. It is best to start with step 1 and work through all the steps at a pace you feel comfortable with. As with any new skill, we should only move on when we feel relatively confident we can manage each step. A good rule of thumb is to move up a step when we can manage it for about five days in a week, and to move back a step if we are struggling for two or three days in a row.

This chapter will take you through the first two steps of the programme; the next chapter will cover the remaining four.

## Step 1: Establishing a regular eating pattern

We will start with establishing a pattern of eating regularly, because this is a good basis for all the other changes we will introduce. Regular eating patterns tend to reduce the body's urge to overeat and help to balance out high and low levels of blood sugar, which have a powerful influence on our appetite and moods.

If you're going to eat regularly, then obviously this means regulation! And yes, there are five rules for you follow. If you have struggled with overeating for some time, you'll probably need to stick to these for a while. They are:

- Plan when you are going to eat.

- Eat by the clock.

- Eat every three to four hours.

- Do not skip an eating episode.

- Do not add an eating episode.

These rules may look a bit daunting at first, even a little authoritarian, and perhaps impossible to stick to. But don't worry: it may take you a little time to establish them, but most people do manage over time. Of course, you may need to bend the rules occasionally – but the more quickly you can establish a regular eating pattern, the easier it will be to stop overeating.

At this point, you are not aiming to change the amounts or types of food that you eat, just to space out your eating more.

To set out your eating plan and record how you keep to it, you will need to use the eating diary that we first saw in Chapter 8. As we discussed earlier, reviewing our diaries can unintentionally lead us into a dieting or self-critical mindset. So do be aware of this potential obstacle and prepare yourself to overcome it by ensuring that you plan your eating and review your diary with your compassionate mind. Begin by engaging your soothing system using your soothing breathing rhythm. When you are ready, bring your compassionate self or compassionate image to mind. Focus on your compassionate feelings of wisdom and encouragement throughout this next exercise, which will take you through reviewing your eating diary to drawing up a regular eating plan.

### Exercise 12.1: Planning to eat more regularly

Start by looking at one day's diary from the perspective of your compassionate mind. Pick a 'typical day' – not one of your worst days for overeating, nor one when you are dieting. What do you notice about the times that you eat? Are there gaps between the times when you eat of more than three to four hours? Or do you find it difficult to leave gaps in your eating – for example, do you eat every couple of hours, or even find yourself grazing all day? If you notice either of these trends, try to use your compassionate self or image to explore these key questions. You can use your compassionate eating formulation and your analysis of overeating and the three emotion regulation systems from Chapter 9 to help you. Always keep in mind that your answers need to come from a perspective of genuinely trying to understand, and kindly and gently support yourself in exploring and making changes in your eating.

## Key questions for planning regular eating

- Why don't I space the meals I eat?

- How does it help me to eat more (or less) frequently than my body needs?

- Would I encourage other people in my life whom I care about to space their eating the way that I do?

- How could I encourage myself to eat more regularly? What could I do or say to help me do this?

When you feel ready, try to develop a daily eating plan based upon the amount and types of food you currently eat. The aim is to break this down into between five and seven eating episodes during the day. Try to eat every three and a half to four hours, starting with breakfast within about thirty minutes of getting up, and ending with a light snack just before you go to bed. You can use Worksheet 11 to set out your eating plan.

Again, you can use your compassionate mind to help you with this. Draw on its wisdom to help you set realistic and achievable expectations about when you are going to eat. It will understand that in these early stages you may still feel the need to overeat and will not expect you to give this up until you are ready. So at this stage if you still need to overeat, for example to help you manage a difficult feeling, that's OK. However, try to do this in a more planned way. For example, you may really want a big tub of ice cream as a comfort food. Instead of coming home and raiding the fridge an hour before you have planned to eat, try to delay your urge and have your ice cream at a time when you have scheduled a meal and when your body is likely to be hungry.

Figure 12.1 shows an example from Alison's regular eating plan, based on the day's diary that we explored earlier. As you can see, she did not reduce the amount that she ate, just changed how it was spaced out. This gave her a greater sense of control over her eating, and also helped her to learn to tolerate her urges to overeat in the knowledge that she could still do this if she needed to but at a time that felt more within her control. We also

**Worksheet 11: Daily meal plan sheet**

| Meal or snack | Time and place | Food and drink to be taken | Comments, including any problems in keeping to meal plan, any solutions to these problems or changes to the plan |
|---|---|---|---|
| Breakfast | | | |
| Mid-morning snack | | | |
| Lunch | | | |
| Mid-afternoon snack | | | |
| Evening meal | | | |
| Evening snack | | | |
| Supper | | | |

| Meal or snack | Time and place | Food and drink to be taken | Comments, including any problems in keeping to meal plan, any solutions to these problems or changes to the plan |
|---|---|---|---|
| Breakfast | Get up at 7 a.m.<br>Eat at 7.30 a.m.<br>With partner | Cereal and milk<br>2 slices of toast<br>Cup of tea | |
| Mid-morning snack | 10.30 a.m.<br>At my desk at work, talking to colleague | Cup of tea<br>5 ginger biscuits | |
| Lunch | 1 p.m.<br>At burger bar, with colleague | Burger meal and milk shake | |
| Mid-afternoon snack | 4.30 p.m.<br>At work, in staff room with other members of staff | Cup of tea<br>5 ginger biscuits | |
| Evening meal | 7.15 p.m.<br>At home with partner<br>At the dinner table | Takeaway meal<br>Individual tub of ice cream<br>2 glasses of wine with meal | |
| Evening snack | 10.30 p.m.<br>At home with partner, watching TV | 5 ginger biscuits<br>2 glasses of wine during the rest of the evening | |
| Supper | No supper as going to bed early | | |

**Figure 12.1:** Alison's meal plan sheet

based the timing of her eating on the hours she was awake. As she got up at 7 a.m. and went to bed at 10.30 p.m., Alison had only one evening snack, which meant she had to space all of her eating across six episodes. However, this was still in the target range of five to seven episodes.

As you can see, Alison also drank the same amount of alcohol on this day too. Clearly, drinking four glasses of wine every night wouldn't be very healthy; however, Alison only drank on one evening a week, and this particular evening was the one night in the week that she spent time with her partner watching a film. Alison acknowledged that she would rather drink less, and over time she managed to space her drinking a little more across the week, while still keeping well within recommended limits. However, in the early stages of learning to eat regularly she did not think she could do this and change her 'drinking for fun and relaxation' at the same time. This is not uncommon, and it is always important to use your compassionate mind to guide how far you can go with making changes at any one time.

You may also notice that Alison made changes not only in when she ate, but also in where she ate. She had noticed that eating alone placed her at greater risk of overeating, and also left her quite vulnerable to the waves of emotion that often accompanied eating. She found that planning to eat in company more helped to provide her with some emotional support (even though the people she ate with at work were unaware that they did this) and also helped to distract her from very self-critical thoughts she had when she was eating.

Interestingly, Alison found that this level of planning took away a lot of her anxiety about eating, and gave her a greater sense of control over her appetite. It also helped her to recognize how different mindsets during the day influenced her and how the people she was with could also affect her urges to eat.

Regular eating on its own can have a positive impact on overeating for some people, so as you start working on this you may want to look back over your diary each week to see if your eating has improved.

Some people find it difficult to establish a regular eating plan. This is not surprising given the obstacles that can arise from have to rearrange when and how we eat, let alone the emotional reasons for eating in the way we have got used to doing. The next exercise is designed to help you explore any blocks you may have to eating regularly and to develop a plan and alternative compassionate thoughts to help you address them.

### EXERCISE 12.2: MANAGING BLOCKS TO EATING REGULARLY

The first step is to imagine that you are going to start eating regularly from tomorrow. This can be quite exciting, as it is a practical start to addressing your overeating; however, you might have a lot of 'yes, buts' or imagine the problems that might arise when you start. These problems could be practical (e.g. 'I don't have food in the house') or related to your thoughts and feelings (e.g. 'I am worried that if I can't comfort eat I won't be able to cope'). Write them down in the left-hand column of Worksheet 12.

The next step is to use your compassionate mind to help you. Take a little time to feel compassion for yourself, either from 'you at your best' or from your compassionate image. Then allow yourself to feel compassion for the blocks that you may encounter in making these changes. Remember, it is not your fault that these blocks arise: maybe there are very real obstacles in the way of you making changes, or maybe thinking of making these changes has activated your threat system in some way and raising obstacles is your brain's way of trying to protect you from harm. Take a little time to explore why these blocks may have arisen and perhaps try to write the reasons for your blocks down too, underneath the blocks themselves on the worksheet.

Finally, imagine how you would feel if you could work though these blocks and manage the feelings that might arise as you did so. You may then wish to add in the right-hand column of the worksheet anything that you could do or say to yourself to help you overcome these blocks and begin to eat regularly.

| Practical and emotional blocks to managing regular eating | Compassionate things I can say to myself or do to help me manage regular eating |
|---|---|
| People are always snacking at work and it is difficult to say no to the biscuits or if they bring chocolates in. They might not like me if I refuse. | This is difficult, as eating is a very sociable thing, especially since I have never tried to say no. But I could choose to try to say no. Other people at work do and people don't think badly of them. I can try to do this one day at a time and see how I feel. |
| I get so peckish – especially if I see things on TV. | This very understandable. I do tend to get peckish a lot in the evening, sometimes because I have not eaten as often as my body needs. Eating more regularly might make this a bit easier. TV is designed to make us peckish, after all – otherwise why make adverts! However, before reaching for that unplanned snack, I can take a breath or two and bring on my compassionate smile and image, and consider how I would feel if I resisted. |
| I am so busy I don't really stop for lunch – well, few people in the office do. | This is hard – especially when other people at work don't stop. However, I do deserve the time to eat and I will try to reschedule my work so that I can. Perhaps I could even encourage a few other people to join me. |

**Figure 12.2   Managing blocks to regular eating: an example**

There is a completed example of the worksheet to help you in Figure 12.2.

When you begin to space your meals out more regularly, you may find that this too can be difficult at times, or that it may provoke painful thoughts and feelings. Keep a note of these difficulties in your eating diary, as when you review your diary these notes will help you understand what works in favour of your eating more regularly and what tends to obstruct you.

*Remember: you are likely to have setbacks along the way. Each new block you that encounter is a sign not of failure, but of your courage in making changes, and an opportunity for you to learn more about how your eating works.*

**Worksheet 12: Managing blocks to regular eating**

| Practical or emotional block to managing regular eating | Compassionate things I can say to myself or do to get past the block |
|---|---|
|  |  |
|  |  |
|  |  |
|  |  |
|  |  |
|  |  |

## *Step 2: Compassionately reducing trigger foods to overeating*

The next step towards your new way of eating is to reduce your risk of being tempted to overeat out of habit or as a way of managing your feelings. The compassionate element here is to work out what you can actually manage without triggering your dieting mind, being overwhelmed by feelings, or depriving yourself of these foods as a way of punishing yourself. This step can be trickier than it looks, but it has the advantage of not requiring you to count calories or plan your meals.

The first thing to do is to identify the types of foods that are most likely to put you at risk of overeating. These may be foods that you associate with comfort eating, or foods that you really enjoy but find it hard to stop eating once you've started.

Returning to Alison's diary, we can see that she had several foods that were associated with emotional comfort (e.g. ginger biscuits) and some foods that she really enjoyed (e.g. burgers or pizza). Some of these foods (e.g. burgers) fell into both categories, in that she enjoyed them and also ate them to 'treat' herself for having been upset. Sometimes Alison would eat sweets when she felt angry with herself. This didn't really give her comfort, and she didn't really enjoy them either. After a while she realized that she ate these sweets when she felt very self-critical because she knew they were 'bad' for her, and she felt she didn't deserve to eat more healthily or to be happy – in other words, these foods became ways of punishing herself. Of course, this was something she really needed to work on, and gradually she managed to stop doing this as she became less self-critical and more self-compassionate.

You can use your own eating diary to work out the types of food that put you at risk of overeating. You can then list them using Worksheet 13, putting them into one or more of the four categories according to why you tend to eat too much of them. Again, Figure 12.3 gives you an example of how to do this using Alison's observations from her diaries.

**Worksheet 13: High-risk foods for overeating**

| Food | Comfort food? Yes/No | Enjoyable food? Yes/No | Treat food? Yes/No | Self-punishing food? Yes/No |
|------|------|------|------|------|
|  |  |  |  |  |
|  |  |  |  |  |
|  |  |  |  |  |
|  |  |  |  |  |
|  |  |  |  |  |
|  |  |  |  |  |
|  |  |  |  |  |
|  |  |  |  |  |
|  |  |  |  |  |
|  |  |  |  |  |
|  |  |  |  |  |
|  |  |  |  |  |
|  |  |  |  |  |
|  |  |  |  |  |
|  |  |  |  |  |
|  |  |  |  |  |
|  |  |  |  |  |
|  |  |  |  |  |
|  |  |  |  |  |
|  |  |  |  |  |

| Food | Comfort food? Yes/No | Enjoyable food? Yes/No | Treat food? Yes/No | Self-punishing food? Yes/No |
|---|---|---|---|---|
| Ginger biscuits | Yes | Not really | No | No |
| Burger | No | Yes | Yes | No |
| Pizza | No | Yes | Yes | No |
| Sweets | No | No | No | Yes |
| Wine | No | Yes | Yes | No |
| | | | | |
| | | | | |
| | | | | |
| | | | | |
| | | | | |
| | | | | |
| | | | | |
| | | | | |
| | | | | |
| | | | | |
| | | | | |
| | | | | |
| | | | | |

**Figure 12.3:** Alison's high-risk foods for overeating

Next, you can begin to work on reducing the amounts of these foods that you eat. Try doing this in four stages.

## 1 Don't tell yourself you are not allowed to have them

This is really important. Humans have a tendency to want what they can't have the minute they are told they can't have it! Remember back in Chapter 3, when I asked you to imagine I'd said you couldn't go to the toilet until you'd finished reading the chapter . . . ?

This urge to do whatever we're told we can't do becomes even stronger if we feel we are denying ourselves something really important to us, such as something we enjoy, or something that gives us comfort, or even something that punishes us. Again, the kinder we are to ourselves about these urges, the easier it is to manage them.

## 2 Work out what the minimum amount of this type of food is that you can eat

The key here is not to stop eating this food entirely. You may still have the need to comfort eat for some time, and will still want to eat many foods because you enjoy them. As you work on changing your eating habits and learn new ways to deal with your feelings, you will also be gradually working on changing the emotional meaning of foods – particularly foods you habitually use to comfort or punish yourself. However, at this stage we are trying to help you reduce the amount of these foods that you eat and at the same time to learn to tolerate your feelings.

To begin with, work out how much of the food you need to eat to get the emotional response that you want. Aim to have only this much of the food available to you at any one time. Of course, you may be tempted to buy more when it has gone. However, this approach will at least mean that you have time to stop and think before you do, so that you can understand your urges and give yourself some time to work with them.

## 3   Gradually reduce the amount of this type of food and learn to tolerate your emotions

The aim here is to allow yourself enough of the food to take the edge off your emotions, but to learn to tolerate them a little more.

To see how this works in practice, let's go back to Alison. Alison found that that ten biscuits tended to be enough for her to feel comforted, and after this she did not feel any more comfort from the biscuits, even if she ate another twenty. So initially she decided to keep ten comfort biscuits that she could use if she needed them. She could only have ten, so that meant that the rest of the packet got thrown away. It was a waste of money, but she would have wasted her money on extra biscuits anyway as they did not provide her with extra comfort, and overeating by eating them all did not stop her eating again later.

After several weeks of doing this Alison felt that she could gradually reduce her reliance on biscuits for emotional comfort. So she decided to reduce the total by one biscuit at a time. Alison managed to do this, and although she felt some distress when she did not have as many biscuits as usual, she felt she could cope as long as she had her safety net of a smaller number of biscuits.

The extent and rate at which you reduce your comfort eating and switch to a healthier balance of foods will be personal to you. People do vary on this, and working out your own way is very important. It is also important to bear in mind that even when we are eating in a more balanced way we are still allowed to eat and enjoy foods that we have used as comfort foods in the past; the key is just to change our relationship with them so they are not used to manage our emotional life. We'll be looking more at learning to enjoy food in a balanced way in the next chapter.

## 4   Increase the delay between the urge to eat your specific food and eating it

This is similar to reducing your intake slowly, in that you are learning to sit with your feelings for a time and finding other ways to manage them.

You may recall that we explored mindfulness in Chapter 5. This is a good time to become more mindful by learning to notice what your feelings are – not to change them, necessarily, but to notice them.

You might also find it useful to write your feelings down. What is going on for you when you turn away from comfort eating or say 'no' to those foods you love? Rather than eating your feelings away you will have written compassionately about them, helping you to understand your feelings better and becoming kinder and gentler with them. You may also find that writing about your feeling lowers the power of the eating urges.

Alison did not feel she could give up biscuits as a comfort food entirely, so when she got down to seven biscuits she worked instead on delaying when she would eat them. Initially she decided that she could only manage one minute of feeling distressed before she ate her biscuits. Gradually she built this up to five minutes, which gave her time to put other coping strategies in place.

The key issue here is learning to become mindful of what we eat and why we eat it. Minimizing the amount of these foods and delaying when you eat them can help you be more in control of the quantity you eat, but more importantly gives you time to reflect on your reason for overeating.

If you eat to treat yourself or because you enjoy a particular type of food, by all means let yourself have these feelings. But if you do, take time over the taste, texture and smell of the food rather than gobbling it down. Make time to eat it in a way that is within your control, and only eat the amount you need to eat to have these feelings.

You may have heard someone call chocolate their 'guilty pleasure'. If you feel like this about, say, chocolate, you could work on reducing the feelings of guilt so that chocolate becomes something you can eat and enjoy. You may well find that you get more satisfaction and enjoyment from one chocolate that you eat slowly, focusing on savouring the taste and texture, than you get from eating a whole box while watching TV! What's happening here is that the feeling of being a naughty child has changed to that of being an adult, in control, who is allowed to feel pleasure.

## SUMMARY

This chapter has explored the first practical steps that you can take towards changing your eating habits. We have explored how you can begin to eat more regularly, and ways to think about and address some of the potential obstacles to this. We have also explored how you can allow yourself to slowly reduce the types and amount of food that can trigger your overeating. These first steps can help you to manage some of the biological highs and lows that come with chaotic eating patterns, and to tolerate and understand your urges to overeat.

The key here is to be compassionate with your attempts to eat more regularly and your urges to overeat. When you feel that you can manage a regular eating pattern, and have a little more control over and understanding of the foods that can trigger overeating, you are ready to move towards the second phase of addressing overeating: changing the amounts and types of food that you eat, and learning to respond to your body's needs. We will look at these steps in the next chapter.

# 13 Towards a new way of eating: the final steps

In Chapter 12 we worked through the first two steps of a programme to establish new and better balanced eating habits: spacing your eating and reducing your intake of foods that are likely to lead to overeating. In this chapter we will move on to cover the remaining four steps: planning what you eat to meet your energy needs; improving the nutritional balance in what you eat; learning to respond to your body's signals for hunger and fullness; and finally, learning to enjoy eating and caring for your body's needs.

## The benefits of meal planning

Meal planning can be tricky to begin with, and I am often asked whether the effort is worth it. It does take some time, certainly, but in my experience meal planning is crucial to resolving overeating. Most people who don't overeat tend to eat regularly, and have a good idea of the types and amount of food they will eat and when. If you don't have a 'sense' of this – and many people who overeat don't – then it's certainly worth learning to acquire it, which is what meal planning is all about.

It is important to recognize that meal planning is not an end in itself. None of us wants to have to plan exactly what we are going to eat and when we will eat it for the rest of our lives! Meal planning is the basis for helping you separate emotional overeating (because you're – for example – angry) from biologically driven overeating (because you're hungry). It can also:

- give us clear idea of what we intend to eat;

- provide a structure to eating;

- help avoid chaotic eating patterns;

- match our energy intake to our energy needs so we are less likely to be hungry;

- give us a baseline from which to make changes in the types and amount of food we eat;

- help us take into account changes in our daily energy needs;

- help us identify and work with times when we eat 'off-plan';

- retrain our body to experience feeling hungry and feeling full.

You are likely to need to plan your eating for between three and six months. Gradually you will develop a menu of foods that you can eat regularly that will meet your nutritional needs and won't lead to overeating – this will make planning (and shopping!) a lot easier – and then move towards eating in response to the signals your body gives you, rather than according to your plan. Please remember that your meal plan should be based around foods that you enjoy, help you feel full, and keep you healthy.

## Potential problems with meal planning

Many people encounter problems in developing a meal plan and putting it into practice.

These may include:

- not knowing how much of a particular food to eat;

- feeling too constrained by the plan;

- difficulty keeping to the plan when other people are around;

- difficulty keeping to the plan when on holiday or visiting others.

It's useful to identify any problems you think might crop up and have some ideas about how to deal with them before you actually start on your meal plan. The next exercise will help you to do this.

EXERCISE 13.1: IDENTIFYING POTENTIAL PROBLEMS WITH MEAL PLANNING

List any problems that you think you might face if you were going to set up a meal plan, and write them in the spaces below.

- 
- 
- 
- 
- 

Now write these in the left-hand column of Worksheet 14. Then, using your compassionate mind to guide you, as you did when you started to plan eating regularly, think about what you might do or say to yourself to overcome these problems and write your suggestions in the right-hand column of the worksheet. Figure 13.1 shows a sample completed worksheet that may help you.

Meal planning is a 'live and learn' process, and we're all likely to come up against a number of challenges to keeping to our plan as we go. No one's expecting you to keep to your meal plan all of the time; that would be unrealistic for any of us! The key is to stick to it as much as possible. That way it can serve its purpose as a way of re-training your body to eat what it needs to eat and when it needs to eat it, and to help you identify the various influences that lead to overeating so you can work on them.

## Step 3: Balancing your energy needs

The first thing to do in drawing up a meal plan is balance your energy needs so that you are eating approximately the amount of calories your body is going to use up.

However, first a word of caution. There's quite a high risk that putting this step into action may trigger your dieting mindset. If your overeating has led to weight gain, you're likely to lose some weight as you establish a better energy balance. It's all too easy to become fixed on this as an achievement in itself, or become impatient with the rate of weight loss and try to eat less than our bodies need. Also, if we try to reduce our overeating too rapidly, we run the risk of triggering our famine survival responses described in Chapter 2.

**Worksheet 14: Dealing with blocks to meal planning**

| Practical and emotional blocks to managing a meal plan | Compassionate things I can say to myself or do to help me manage my meal plan |
|---|---|
|  |  |
|  |  |
|  |  |
|  |  |
|  |  |
|  |  |
|  |  |

| Practical and emotional blocks to managing a meal plan | Compassionate things I can say to myself or do to help me manage my meal plan |
|---|---|
| I don't like to plan when and what to eat. | Most people don't like to plan like this. *But* I deserve the opportunity to develop a better relationship with food. I have been able to schedule regular eating a little better. I can live with this for a while to see whether it can help me; if it doesn't I can always stop doing it. |
| Eating to a plan makes me feel controlled, and brings up unhappy memories of the way people fed me in the past. | It is really sad that people were controlled by eating in unhelpful and unkind ways in the past. It is also understandable as overeating and dieting often helps you to feel in control. *But* now I am an adult I can choose to take control of my eating and learn new ways to take control of my life. I don't really control food anyway; it controls me because I can't stop overeating when I want to. |
| I don't know what a normal portion of pizza is. | I can look up what a normal portion is in my calorie-counting book. I can work out how many calories of pizza I am going to eat as part of my evening meal and allow myself this. |
| The plan does not give me any freedom. | If I give myself too much freedom I know I will overeat. It is worth having some constraints to help me work out why I overeat. I can choose what I eat on the plan. |
| It's hard to keep to the plan when other people are around. | Everyone struggles to eat consistently when they are with others. I can plan in advance for the kind of meal other people might eat. I can use this as a chance to practise saying no when people offer me food. |

**Figure 13.1:** Dealing with blocks to meal planning: an example

So here are some guidelines to help you manage this step, summarized in four key points:

- Know what your needs are now.

- Know how much you are overeating or undereating by.

- Don't reduce your energy intake too quickly.

- Plan your eating at least one day in advance.

## Know what your needs are now

We explored our energy and nutritional needs in some detail in Chapter 11. You can use this information as the basis of your meal plan.

## Know how much you are overeating or undereating by

Again, the information you collected in Chapter 11 will help you to calculate this. Remember to look at these needs day to day as well as across the week to avoid the urge to overeat that comes from trying to 'make up' for overeating on the previous day.

## Don't reduce your intake too quickly

Most of us will be familiar with the notion that diets would only aim to reduce our weight by 1–2 lb (0.5–1 kg) a week. The evidence suggests that this is the most our body can manage healthily. If you tend to overeat as a consequence of getting caught up in a dieting mindset when you start to reduce the amount you're eating, even this may be too much. Ideally, you might aim at reducing your overall energy intake by about 200 calories a day until it roughly matches your daily energy needs and so you are in a neutral energy balance.

Remember, changing your eating is a long-term process, and the goal is to make changes that will last as part of a healthier relationship with food, eating and your body. This is a little easier if we aim to make smaller, but sustainable, changes in our eating.

## Plan your eating at least one day in advance

This does require some forward thinking, and you may find it difficult at first; but over time you will get used to having a range of options of foods you enjoy and that meet your energy needs so that you can ring the changes from day to day without having to start from scratch every time.

The principles of drawing up a meal plan are basically the same as those you used to establish a regular eating pattern in the previous chapter, and you can use a similar form to set out your plan. This is provided in Worksheet 15 (there are more copies of the worksheet at the back of the book, and you can copy as many as you need – or make your own). The only change is that now, as well as eating regularly, you're planning what and how much you will eat to roughly balance your eating intake with your needs.

So meal planning has the same five rules as for planning regular eating, with two more new ones (in italics in the list):

- Plan when you are going to eat.

- *Plan how much you are going to eat at each episode.*

- Eat by the clock.

- Eat every three to four hours.

- Do not skip an eating episode.

- Do not add an eating episode.

- *Drink enough fluid (about 8 glasses, or 2 litres) a day.*

In Figure 13.2 you will find a sample day's meal plan to guide you.

## Step 4: Developing a healthy nutritional balance

Sometimes when we begin to plan our meals we can also begin to change the types of food we eat. However, many of us find this a step too far at first, which is why Step 3 above simply concentrated on planning how much and when you will eat. Once you have established your meal plan, however, and are getting used to aiming at a neutral energy balance, the next step is to work at getting a better nutritional balance as well. You can use the information in Chapter 11 (especially Table 11.1 and Figure 11.1, the 'eatwell plate') to guide you on proportions of the various food types.

One of the problems that can arise with doing this is that we are often brought up to associate healthy eating with boring meals, or feeling forced to eat foods we don't like. The key to improving our nutritional balance is to explore a wider range of foods. This may mean that we need to experiment a little more. For example, you might think you don't like the taste of vegetables – but there are an awful lot of different vegetables, and maybe you were put off by just one or two, perhaps always cooked the same way. So you may need to try a lot of different types, cooked and prepared in quite a lot of ways, before you can really decide what you like.

This can be quite an exciting time in your process of tackling overeating. Here are a few tips you might want to try to help you.

- Use your meal plan and the information in Chapter 11 to explore how your current eating fits with a nutritionally balance food intake.

- Try to make small changes in your balance and then build on them. For example, you may want to increase your intake of fruit and vegetables by 100 calories a day at first, swapping this number of calories for another food type (perhaps reducing sugary or higher-fat foods by the same amount).

- Have some fun experimenting with food. For example, you might write the names of twenty types of fruit on pieces of paper, mix them up and pick one at random. Go and find one of whatever it is. If you really don't like it, try something else.

- Experiment with cooking food as well. For example, my kids really don't like carrot that much, so my wife mashes it with potato.

- Learn what you like and don't like; and don't eat what you don't like!

## Step 5: Learning to respond to feelings of hunger and fullness

Meal planning is designed to help us retrain our eating patterns so that we can then move on to deciding what and when to eat on the basis of whether our body feels hungry or full, rather than on the basis of our habits and

**Worksheet 15: Tomorrow's meal plan**

| Day and date | | |
|---|---|---|
| Eating episode | Time | Food and drink to be taken (including type and amount) |
| Breakfast | a.m. | |
| Mid-morning snack | a.m. | |
| Lunch | p.m. | |
| Mid-afternoon snack | p.m. | |

| Evening meal | p.m. | | Supper | p.m. | |
|---|---|---|---|---|---|
| | | | | | |

**Monday 30 March**

| Eating episode | Time | Food and drink to be taken (including type and amount)<br>Please note: where there is a choice of portion sizes (e.g. 2 or 3 potatoes), women should have the smaller size portion (e.g. 2 potatoes) and men the larger one (e.g. 3 potatoes). | |
|---|---|---|---|
| Breakfast | 7.30 a.m. | STARCH | 1 bowl cereal<br>2 slices bread |
| | | FAT/SUGAR | butter or margarine<br>jam, honey or marmalade |
| Mid-morning snack | 10.30 a.m. | DAIRY | 1 yoghurt (not diet) |
| | | FRUIT | 1 apple |
| Lunch | 1.00 p.m. | STARCH | 2 slices bread or average baked potato |
| | | FATS | mayonnaise, butter, margarine or salad cream |
| | | PROTEIN | 1–2 slices meat, or 2 eggs or 2 oz cheese or tinned fish or 1 small tin baked beans<br>(men should double these amounts – i.e. 2 full sandwiches or 2 baked potatoes) |
| | | VEG. | salad if wanted |
| | | DAIRY | 2 scoops of ice cream |
| Mid-afternoon snack | 4.30 p.m. | FRUIT | 1 banana<br>1 fruit juice |

| Evening meal | 8 p.m. | STARCH | 2–3 medium potatoes or 4–6 heaped tablespoons of cooked rice or pasta or 2–3 slices bread |
| | | FATS | oil in cooking or butter or margarine or mayonnaise or salad cream |
| | | PROTEIN | 2 slices meat or 2 eggs or 2 oz cheese or small tin baked beans or average serving fish or 4 fish fingers |
| | | VEG | vegetables or salad |
| | | SUGAR | 1 chocolate-covered biscuit |
| Supper | 11 p.m. | DAIRY (men should add an extra snack) | milky drink |

**Figure 13.2:** Sample daily meal plan

emotions. Within the structure of regular, balanced eating that your meal plans provide, you will gradually learn to experience these feelings of hunger and fullness. A healthier nutritional balance will mean that most of the calories we eat come from the types of food that are most likely to help us feel full and satisfied.

Some diets will have trained your body to respond to fluid as if it were food, for example by getting you to drink a lot before you eat. Interestingly, a recent study has shown that this doesn't really work that well at a biological level, as our body recognizes the energy content of food, not simply the volume in our stomachs. However, drinking too much before you eat can make it more difficult for you to work out whether you are full or not, so at first you may find it easier to drink when you have finished eating.

Often the ways in which we eat can obscure our natural feelings of hunger or fullness or lead us to ignore our body's signals. To become aware of them again we may need to learn to be more mindful of the experience of eating. If we think about which Western countries have the longest lifespan and most healthy lifestyles, we tend to think of the countries of southern Europe and the 'Mediterranean' diet. This is based around fresh fruit and vegetables, starchy food such as pasta, and protein from meat and fish.

However, this is only part of the story. The 'Mediterranean diet' is also associated with a very specific way of eating. Eating tends to be a shared family ritual, each dish is savoured, and a meal can last for several hours – including the occasional glass of wine, also sipped and savoured rather than gulped down. This is in fact the very type of eating we evolved for. The key point is that food is not just fuel that we eat in front of the TV, at our desks or workstations, or even behind the steering wheel. Allowing ourselves to eat more slowly, to savour the tastes and textures of food, and to begin to digest one course before we decide whether we want the next one, can all help us listen to our body and become more sensitive to its signals.

You can add this step at any stage of your journey to a new way of eating. However, the reason I have put it here, towards the end of the six-step programme, is that if your eating has become entangled with managing difficult feelings, then being more in touch with feelings of hunger and fullness may also put you in touch with difficult emotional experiences or memories. If this is the case for you, it can be helpful to eat in a *less* mindful way in the early stages of changing your eating. Nevertheless, to beat overeating for good we do need to become more mindful when we are eating or when we have the urge to eat. You can use your eating diary to help you note down any thoughts and feelings that you have when you eat more mindfully.

If you feel ready to embark on this step, start by becoming more mindful of the physical experience of hunger, so you can begin to use this as a guide to when to eat and how much you need. Sometimes it is easier to recognize when we have eaten far too much than when we are hungry. So to begin with, spend a little time remembering the last time this happened. How did your body feel? When did you notice that you had eaten too much? What happened that helped you to ignore these feelings of becoming full while you were still eating?

Next you may want to think about the last time you were so extremely hungry that you found it really hard to stop eating once you had started. How did this feel in your body? What things had led you to ignore your hunger this much?

Finally, think about the last time you felt you had eaten just enough to feel satisfied (a bit like Goldilocks and her porridge – you got it just right!). This is the sensation that you want to experience to guide you in knowing when your body has had enough to eat. Sometimes we will not get this absolutely right – we will have eaten just a little too much or remain just a bit hungry.

Again, using your compassionate mind, try to bring to mind each of these stages, and explore how it felt and what helped you to notice when you had eaten enough or just slightly more than your body needed.

You can practise this skill by rating your hunger and fullness, and we will explore this in the next exercise.

## EXERCISE 13.2: LEARNING TO FEEL HUNGER AND FULLNESS

In this exercise you can work on becoming more mindful of your body's hunger and fullness signals.

To begin with, make a note every time you eat of how hungry you feel before you eat and how full you feel after you eat. You could do this in your eating diary or meal plan, if you're still keeping one.

When you have a better idea of how hungry and full you are before and after you eat, you can move on to the next stage, which is to track these sensations during the day, and when you are actually eating.

As you develop this skill, you can then use the knowledge you gain to decide when you need to eat and when you have had enough to eat. It can also be helpful to make a note of whether other things interfere with your ability to keep an eye on (and respond to) your body's needs – for example, feeling tired, angry or upset, or becoming too engrossed in other activities.

You can use the following rating scales to help you. The 'hungriness scale' is something you can use throughout the day, perhaps keeping a note of your score every hour or so and every time you eat. If you use it together with your eating diary it can help you to explore any things that increase your hunger. These may include the desire to eat that is triggered by changes in your blood sugar levels when you need food; however, you may also notice associations between certain feelings (such as tiredness or anger) and increased feelings of hunger. The 'fullness scale' is designed to be used while you are eating: perhaps just keep a note of changes in feelings of fullness during your meal and for around thirty minutes after you finish eating.

### Hungriness scale

1 = Extremely hungry – so much so that you will find it very hard to stop eating when you are full or that you can't wait for your next meal.

2 = Moderately hungry – you may still be inclined to overeat or to snack a little before your next meal.

3 = Slightly hungry – you may have strong urges to overeat or snack and have to work hard to resist.

4 = Ready to eat – you know you are ready for your next meal but don't have a strong urge to snack and are unlikely to overeat when you have it.

5 = Don't need to eat – you don't feel hungry and if you were to eat now you would feel overfull.

### Fullness scale

1 = Not full at all – you are still hungry after your meal and are very likely to overeat.

2 = Moderately full – you are still a bit hungry and want to carry on eating; you may end up overeating.

3 = Full and satisfied – you have eaten enough to feel full and don't want to eat any more.

4 = Overfull – you have eaten more than enough, perhaps eating a few bites more than you need.

5 = Far too full – you feel very uncomfortable with the amount you have eaten, perhaps bloated, even physically unwell.

Ideally, we want to start eating as soon as we start feeling hungry (4 on the hungriness scale) and stop when we reach 3 on the fullness scale, so that we will not overeat. You may need to spend some time learning to do this, as we can all get a little out of touch with our body's needs; the key is to try to avoid getting so detached from what your body is telling you that you end up getting very hungry and then overeating as a result. It is also important to remember that your body tends to take a little while to give you signals that you are full; so eating more slowly with fewer distractions is really important at this stage, so you can become aware of feelings of fullness gradually growing.

## What am I hungry for?

Recently I had an interesting discussion with a dietitian colleague of mine who regularly asks her clients an interesting question in relation to eating more mindfully: What are you hungry *for*? Now, as a psychologist I thought she meant: What emotional needs is your eating helping you with? – and of course this is an important aspect of this work. However, this wasn't quite what she had meant, and what she said was fascinating. She is interested in our body's intuitive wisdom in knowing what it needs and hungering for that thing; sometimes, she said, we need to know what this is in order for our body to feel satisfied. The most extreme example of this can be some of the curious food cravings that happen during pregnancy. But let's take a more everyday example. Let's imagine you really want some orange-flavoured chocolate, but deny yourself this and have an orange instead. My guess is that no matter how many oranges you eat you will still be 'hungry' for the chocolate. Being aware of this can help you to recognize what it is you want and then be satisfied with a little of it, rather than spending so much time denying your needs that you eat food you don't want and then, having denied yourself and so increased the craving, end up overeating the thing you wanted in the first place!

## Step 6: Learning to enjoy food again

This is your final step along the road to a new way of eating. By this stage you should be able to keep (mostly) to your meal plans and/or be more in touch with your body's needs. You will also be able to recognize 'trigger foods' and other things that are likely to lead to overeating.

You may also have included in your planned eating some of the foods that you enjoy. However, some foods that you used to enjoy may now have less pleasant associations. For example, you may like the taste of cakes, but have learned to be afraid of the consequences of eating them. Or you may have always eaten sweets when you overate, but ate so many so fast that you never really knew whether you liked the taste. You may have eaten so much of a particular food that all you associate with it now is the experience of feeling overfull and bloated.

If certain foods have specific unpleasant associations for you, you may wish to start to weaken and break these links so that you can once again allow yourself to enjoy these foods. The next exercise can help you do this.

## Exercise 13.3: Changing food associations

Choose a food that you have previously been concerned about eating but think that you might enjoy, or would like to eat again. Plan to eat some of this food at a time you do not feel hungry. Then bring your soothing system into play by practising your soothing breathing rhythm or safe place imagery. When you feel ready, put a piece of the food in your mouth. Take time to experience the smell, taste and texture of the food. What do you notice? Is the food something that you like? Does eating the food trigger any other experiences, for example unpleasant memories? What might worry you if you allowed yourself to enjoy what you have eaten?

If you notice memories, thoughts and feelings cropping up that could stop you enjoying the food, don't eat any more of it just now but pause and write these down. Now think what your compassionate mind might say or do to help you cope with these thoughts. You could use a version of the compassionate thought balancing form (Worksheet 2) to help you, though of course with new column headings; or you might like to write yourself a compassionate letter (we will be exploring this skill in the next chapter).

When you feel ready, you can repeat the exercise with another piece of the food; but this time, gently and kindly, imagine – or even actually say out loud – these new compassionate thoughts as you are eating. With practice you will learn to associate these new thoughts with these foods and to allow yourself to enjoy them.

As well as returning to foods you used to enjoy, try also to increase the variety of foods that you eat so you can learn that you enjoy exploring new tastes, smells and textures.

Another aspect of learning to enjoy food again is getting used to eating with others. Many people who overeat have come to avoid eating socially, either because they are concerned what other people might think about what they eat (for example, seeing them as greedy) or because they are more likely to overeat in these situations. Again, this is something you can overcome with practice – after all, you deserve to eat out, and to eat with your friends and family, as much as anyone else! This is the time to learn to reclaim eating as a pleasant and normal human social activity that you no longer need to be afraid of. The next exercise will help you to do this.

### EXERCISE 13.4: ENJOYING EATING SOCIALLY

Again you can use the thought balancing form (Worksheet 2), with appropriate column headings. Begin by writing down in the left-hand column any thoughts or feelings that have stopped you, or put you off, eating with other people. Now bring your compassionate mind into play and explore ways in which you could address these concerns from a compassionate perspective. If you have noted that you are concerned about how other people would react to seeing you eat, you might want to think about this from the perspective of your compassionate image; would they see it as fair to stop people eating socially and enjoying food?

Another way to begin feeling more comfortable eating socially is gradually to build up the range of people you eat with or places where you eat. The key word here is 'gradually': for example, you might start by having a meal with just one other person whom you know, like and trust, and then try eating with a small group of just two or three people. This will give you the opportunity to practise your new compassionate thoughts and behaviour. When you feel comfortable in twos and threes, you could then gradually expand the range of people you eat with and places where you eat.

The key to this last step in the programme is to experiment and learn to have fun with foods. Allow yourself to reclaim your relationship with eating, so that you enjoy food, safe in the knowledge that you are in tune with your body's needs and have alternative ways of managing your feelings. It is this feeling of pleasure and safety, rather than the rigid (and impossible) rules of dieting, or the chaos of overeating to manage your feelings or from habit, that will make eating a 'risk free' and enjoyable part of your life.

# Putting it all together: caring for your body with compassion

Our bodies need to be cared for if we are going to get the most out of them, and eating healthily is a big part of this – but it is not the whole story. None of us is going to have the perfect body, and indeed it's an illusory aim. A more realistic aim is to have a body that is healthy for as long as possible, and a body that we appreciate and enjoy. To this end, we need not only to eat well, but also to attend to two other needs: *activity* and *rest*.

## *Physical activity*

Our long-term health has far more to do with how physically fit we are than how much we weigh. The good news is that our evolution means that our bodies are relatively low-maintenance compared to, for example, those of a thoroughbred race horse (or even our pet dogs). We need about one hour of physical activity every day that increases out heart rate and keeps it up, without making us out of breath (a good indicator of this is whether we can still keep up a conversation). It seems that we can even do this in short bursts of five to ten minutes and still get the same health benefits. Sadly, most of us – including me! – don't always do this. We tend to be very sedentary, because of the changes in lifestyle that have come with working longer and longer hours in less physical jobs. Or we engage in intense programmes of activity that we find hard to sustain – typically as a New Year's resolution to join a gym.

Our average levels of physical activity, particularly among younger people, are going down year by year. For a whole range of reasons, people who overeat tend to do even less physical activity than the already unhealthily low average. This is not good for our mental or our physical health. Lack of activity can lead to low mood, tiredness and anxiety, and a range of physical problems, as well as leaving us weighing more than our genetic makeup intended.

However, many of us also overexercise, usually by setting targets for exercise that are not sustainable – for example, vowing that we will go running every day, come rain or shine. We also tend to link exercise with the dieting mindset: we exercise to lose weight, and we give it up when we give up our diet.

So we need to aim for a compassionate level of physical activity that recognizes and is in tune with our body's needs, but that also reflects and responds to our physical health – so that, for example, we don't force ourselves to go running when we are ill. We also need to break the link between 'exercise' and the dieting mindset.

In fact, it can be better not to think of 'exercise' at all, but of 'physical activity' instead. For many of us, formal exercise can have a whole range of negative connections – for example, with being bullied into cross-country running at school, or being humiliated by not being picked for the football or hockey team. For others, exercise simply became 'uncool', and was abandoned as they grew older. Many young girls give up formal physical exercise as they reach their teens for this reason.

Starting formal exercise or taking up sport again can take a lot of courage if we've had any of these types of experience in the past – and it can be even harder if we don't feel good about our fitness levels or our size and shape. Many people can and do find going to the gym or taking up a sport a fun and useful way to increase their physical activity. However, physical activity covers a whole range of things a long way from gym workouts and exercise classes. It can include dancing around at home, going for a walk, gardening – even housework.

The key to increasing your physical activity is to choose a variety of things you're prepared to do now, and a couple you'd like to work towards. Ideally, this will build on things we already do; but remember, variety is the spice of life. An extra hour of housework may increase your activity levels but may not be as much fun as going for a walk with a friend!

Increasing your physical activity will take some planning, and you might want to add it in to your meal planning. If you do this, you can use your increased activity to improve your energy balance – but do bear in mind that activity tends to make us hungry, so we need to plan to eat and replace fluid afterwards.

Start by increasing your physical activity levels slowly: listen to your body, and ease off when it tells you that you're doing too much. Remember, you should still be able to hold a conversation: pushing through pain is not necessary and it's certainly not compassionate. The usual advice also applies: before you begin to increase your activity, check with your doctor that there's no medical reason why you shouldn't.

If you are taking at least an hour's physical activity a day then you are meeting your body's needs. Anything over and above this will affect your energy balance for the day. As you get more in touch with your hunger you are likely to notice this increase in energy need, and to respond to it appropriately.

## Rest

Our body needs time to rest and repair itself just as much as it needs food to fuel it and physical activity to maintain it. We get most of the rest we need when we sleep, but we also need to have some rest during the day, particularly if we have just finished physical activity (and more than usual, of course, if we are unwell).

It is easy to work all day, come home and do housework and look after other people, or even carry on working from home, right up until bedtime. If we don't get enough rest we can end up feeling stressed, anxious, depressed and irritable – all of which can lead to overeating. So we may need to begin to plan in periods of rest during the day, even if it is only a couple of minutes at a time. This can also help us to learn why we don't allow ourselves to rest. It may be that we have just got out of the habit; but it may also be that we keep busy to avoid difficult thoughts and feelings, or because we feel compelled to. You might like to use some of the exercises in Chapter 6 on dealing with blocks to compassion to help you explore and overcome these obstacles to taking rest.

Many people who overeat also have problems with sleeping. Lack of sleep can directly increase our likelihood of overeating. If we are awake for longer periods we have more opportunities for overeating; not having enough sleep also lowers our mood, and leaves us too tired to plan eating and prepare food, or to keep physically active. It can even leave us craving foods to give us an energy burst – usually those high in fat and sugar!

Sleep problems can be a complicated area. However, the following simple 'sleep hygiene' tips can help:

- Always get up at the same time, no matter how tired you are.

- Don't sleep during the day.

- Only go to bed when you are tired.

- Use your bed for sleeping: don't sleep elsewhere, e.g. in a chair or on the sofa.

You may wish to develop a bedtime routine to prepare you for sleep. This could usefully include the following elements:

- Cut out caffeinated drinks (e.g. coffee, tea, cola etc.) for *at least* four hours before bedtime.

- Avoid drinking alcohol for a couple of hours before going to bed.

- Don't overstimulate your mind by doing mentally challenging work, playing computer games or watching scary or upsetting TV programmes for a couple of hours before bedtime.

- Have a milky drink before you go bed.

- Spend a little time getting ready for bed, getting changed into your night clothes, cleaning your teeth etc., to give yourself the message that you are going to sleep soon.

- If you like to read in bed, try to choose something that is not too interesting or emotionally stimulating.

- If you can't sleep after ten minutes, get up and repeat your bedtime ritual until you feel sleepy.

This type of sleeping plan may well leave you feeling exhausted for a week or so, but can be very effective in establishing a sleep routine. We all struggle to get to sleep, or to stay asleep, at times in our lives, but usually this phase passes after a day or two. If you have problems with sleeping that last longer than this, have a word with your doctor. You can also find resources to help you work on this on your own in the 'Useful resources' section at the end of the book.

### SUMMARY

This chapter has taken you through the final steps towards a new way of eating. These include planning your energy balance and nutritional needs, learning to respond to natural feelings of hunger and fullness, and learning to enjoy food again, both on your own and in company. We've also explored how to care for your body in other ways by getting appropriate amounts of activity and rest.

It may be that these practical approaches are enough to help you to stop overeating, or at least to improve how often it happens and how severe it gets. Still, however much we plan, our emotions and thoughts can still get in the way, and may still trigger overeating from time to time even when we have established a better structure to our eating. One way of using your compassionate mind to help you with these troublesome thoughts and feelings is compassionate letter writing. In the next chapter we will explore how to go about this, so that you can use it alongside all the practical skills you have learned over the course of the past chapters.

# 14 Compassionate letter writing

For thousands of years people have found that writing down what they're concerned or worried about can help them 'get it off their chest' and either defuse difficult feelings or put them aside until they are ready to work on them. Writing can be helpful to us for a number of reasons. It slows our thinking down in a way that's difficult to do if we just think in our heads. It helps us to become more reflective and thoughtful. Also, we can read back what we have written, and revisiting our thoughts in this way can give us new insights and ideas about what may help us. In this chapter we are going to focus on a particular approach to writing things down that takes the form of composing a letter to ourselves in a style that offers us support, understanding and kindness to help us deal with the challenges of life. We call this approach *compassionate letter writing*.

In compassion focused therapy we can use letter writing to develop our skills in both offering and receiving compassion. Letters can help us to capture thoughts, feelings, new ways of paying attention and new ways of acting on paper. They can also help us to identify blocks to compassion which can occur in imagery work or when we are trying out new ways of behaving compassionately. Compassionate letter writing can be used in addition to the other skills we have worked on in this book. Ideally, as with each new skill we have learned, we don't want to be trying it for the first time when we are in the grip of another powerful mindset that can lead us to overeat. So, initially at least, we will use our letters as a way of planning to manage overeating in the near future. As you become more skilled you may find that you can use letter writing to help you deal with urges to overeat as they happen, or with other painful emotions or feelings.

We will explore how this kind of writing can help you put together the information and analysis that you have developed about your overeating, and the skills you have learned so far, in a structured way. Many people have found this type of structure very helpful when using their compassionate mind to help them find lasting solutions to overeating.

## Getting started

There is nothing rushed in compassionate letter writing – just take your time. Having said that, once you are ready and in the right frame of mind (more on this below), it's useful to start writing regardless of whether or not you know what you're going to write. In fact, in many ways it's a good idea not to work things out too far in advance but to just 'go with the flow'. Sometimes people sit staring at a blank page, going over and over in their heads what to write. This can be linked to the self-critical or judging mindset, trying to work it all out in advance and make sure you do it 'right'. But there is no right or wrong here, and it's fine to start and stop – you might have a number of false starts before you get into the flow.

What 'getting into the flow' really means is allowing your writing hand rather than your head to do the work, so that you're writing as you think rather than thinking first and then writing. As I say, the biggest block to this is trying to have too much clarity before you start. If you just start writing, regardless of whether what you're putting down seems sensible or indeed makes much sense, then slowly the flow may come.

There is always the temptation to want to write the 'perfect letter'. I never have, nor will I ever, and nor has anyone I have worked with – but that's OK! What we are looking for is a 'good enough' letter to help bring feelings of compassion to the fore and to get us into the compassionate mindset. So you may also need to be compassionate with your inability to do 'the perfect' letter whenever you attempt the exercise! I have been writing compassionate letters for several years, and I still find it a difficult, although incredibly useful, skill to use when I am dealing with challenging events or painful feelings in my own life.

When you feel more comfortable writing letters, it is likely that you will intuitively know what the feelings and challenges are that you want your letter to help you think about and work with. However, many people who overeat can find this difficult to begin with – not least because overeating often helps us manage difficult feelings, and we may be so used to doing this that we're not even aware of precisely what is behind the distress we are trying to soothe by eating. In my experience these roots of distress become a little clearer when we begin thinking about giving up overeating as a way of helping us to manage things. Compassionate letter writing can help you to look at this distress more clearly but also in a way that is manageable, to give you an opportunity to explore your feelings and thoughts. It can enable you to practise bringing your soothing system and compassionate mind together to find new solutions to your difficulties.

## Setting the scene for compassionate letter writing

There are a number of key steps in developing a compassionate letter. Before we even begin to write, it is important that we are in the right frame of mind. To do this you may wish to use your soothing breathing rhythm or the safe place exercise introduced in Chapter 5. If you are feeling really distressed before you start, you might like to use some of the self-soothing exercises we explored in Chapter 6. When you notice your soothing system coming into play, you can then use compassionate imagery to help you.

There are two ways you can use imagery at this point. The first way is to create a compassionate frame of mind within yourself. When you are ready, imagine yourself as a compassionate person and go through the 'you at your best' exercise that we explored in Chapter 5. So you will imagine yourself to have wisdom, strength, confidence and great kindness. Remember to spend time trying to get into this mindset, even if only a little way. Try to create a compassionate expression on your face and to focus on what your tone of your voice would be if you were to speak. Spend a few moments focusing on what it feels like and sounds like to become 'you at your best'.

Alternatively, if you prefer, you can imagine your compassionate companion, that person, being or element that conveys great compassion (involving wisdom, strength and kindness) to you. Remember, you don't have to have a well-defined image; just a presence that you can sense with you, that is focused on your well-being and recognizes the nature of the difficulty you are struggling with, is fine. Imagine the sound of the voice or any communication that comes from them as wise and strong, expressed with great warmth and kindness, never judgemental, always understanding and looking for the helpful way forward.

When you can feel your compassionate mind or compassionate companion is actively with you, you can begin to work though the various steps to letter writing that I have outlined below. Don't feel you have to go right through the process at once; take your time and only go as far as you're comfortable with in one sitting. You will need a bit of time to work on letter writing: it's a good idea to put aside an hour or so each time you try it. The key is not to rush things, to feel comfortable with the skills in each step before you move on to the next. You can use your compassionate mind to help you work out if you are ready to move on, and to offer you support and encouragement while you experiment with this new way of working with your thoughts, feelings and eating.

You may wish to plan for something soothing or distracting to do after you have finished writing your letter, and to allow yourself time and space before and after your writing session to care for yourself.

## Steps to compassionate letter writing

### Step 1: Paying compassionate attention to your feelings

This involves both any difficult feelings that you are experiencing now and any you anticipate experiencing in a new situation. Start by bringing to mind the changes in your eating that you want to make, or the situation or feeling that you want to work on that may trigger overeating in the near future. This is likely to bring your threat or drive system into action. Notice how thinking about this affects the feelings in your body, and the thoughts and emotions that come up. You only need to stay with this focus for a minute or so, perhaps making a few notes of the thoughts, feelings and any physical sensations you notice as you go along. The changes or situation you have in mind will be the focus of your letter, but we don't want to stay with the feelings any longer than we need to work out what our letter is going to help us with. Usually about a minute is enough! As soon as you can feel in touch with this, it is time to move on to the next step.

## Step 2: Stepping outside the feeling

Having noticed with mindful attention the effects that the prospect of changing your eating (or whatever other situation you have in view) has on your threat or drive system, your aim now is to step outside those feelings a little. You can use the soothing breathing rhythm and other mindfulness exercises you have practised to help you to do this. In this way you can experience the emotions that you are struggling with without getting too caught up in them, or feeling the need to act on them immediately.

## Step 3: Experiencing safeness

Of course, if you feel you can tolerate your feelings and move straight into your compassionate image now, you are free to do so. However, if you are finding it difficult to stay with your feelings – for example, if your threat system becomes too active, or your drive system wants you to do something to change your feeling state – then it can be helpful to work on your safe place imagery first. When you notice that your threat system or drive system has dampened down a bit, but you are still aware of the feelings that you may need to work with, then it's a good time to move on to the next step.

## Step 4: Activating your compassionate image

The next step is to bring your mind back to your compassionate image. This could be 'you at your best' or your compassionate companion. You can do this by working through the process described above under 'setting the scene'. It's best not to begin letter writing until you feel confident that you can bring this image to mind, even if only as a fleeting experience.

When we are developing our compassionate image we want to make it as much of an emotional, bodily and sensory experience as we can – even if this is only a fleeting sensation. It may also be helpful to have something with you to look at, or touch, or smell, that reminds you of your image, and helps to keep your soothing system active.

It is the feelings of compassion flowing into us from our image that are so important. We want to try to tone up our soothing system, not just on an intellectual level but also on an emotional level. When you can feel this compassion, then it is time to begin writing your letter.

The key to writing your letter is to write it from the perspective of the compassionate self. The compassionate self understands, empathizes with and supports you unconditionally. It is wise strong, and caring. It will recognize that thinking about doing things differently, or understanding ourselves in new ways, can be painful; so it won't rush your letter, or ask you to make changes that you are not ready for.

It can be difficult to activate our compassionate self, and if you find it tricky, don't worry: this happens to all of us. It may be that this is as far as you can get on your first four or five tries at compassionate letter writing. This is perfectly normal – it can take several weeks, even months, of returning to practice before some people are ready to move on to the next stage of their letter.

## Step 5: Beginning your letter

As someone who has always struggled to write the first paragraph of anything, I know that compassionate letters can be tricky to write. I, and many people I have worked with, have found it helpful to have a structure to follow that gives us some idea of where to begin and where to move on to. So the next steps will set out a suggested sequence of themes that you might follow. For now, we'll start with a couple of general guidelines.

### Recognizing your compassionate qualities

In the first part of your letter it is important to help yourself recognize your own internal wisdom, courage, strength and resilience. This is because we can often feel overwhelmed by our problem or become locked into a very self-critical way of thinking. If we are stuck in these feelings it can be hard to recognize these qualities in ourselves that we will need to help face our problems. So we are aiming at least to remind ourselves that we have these qualities, even if we can't feel them.

## First person (I) or third person (you)?

Sometimes we find it hard to write directly about ourselves in the first person (e.g. 'I have been very brave in acknowledging feeling angry this week and in trying to understand why I feel this way'). So it can help to write your letter in the third person to begin with, ideally as coming from your compassionate self or companion (e.g. 'You have been very brave' etc.). When you feel ready you can then start to write first-person letters.

Imagine for the rest of this chapter that your name is Kerry and that you are writing your first compassionate letter to yourself. So you'll start by writing in the third person, beginning 'Dear Kerry', and then go on to recognize the compassionate, wise, brave, strong and resilient things that you feel that Kerry has done well over the previous week and in the past. At this point you're not focusing particularly on your achievements so much as on the qualities of compassion that you want to foster. This part of the letter should also include your own (or your companion's) compassionate feelings for Kerry. For example:

> *Dear Kerry, it has been very difficult to watch you struggle with your feelings over the past week and it is not surprising that you have ended up overeating. I understand that life has been hard for you in the past, and is hard at the moment. However, I have been impressed by how courageous you have been in trying to tackle these feelings and to understand how your brain and your body work. I have also been impressed by the ways in which you have been able to be caring for others, even though you have been upset, and to carry on with some things at work that you found difficult.*

It is really important to try to think about specific examples that our compassionate image would offer us. You may not even believe your compassionate image at this point, but it is important to activate that part of your brain that focuses on your compassionate capacities, your courage and your ability to tolerate and manage distressing and difficult things.

## Step 6: Empathy and understanding

It is important that our letters allow us to express empathy with and understanding of the struggles that we have experienced in the past, are having now, or may be facing over the coming days or weeks. There are three important elements to this that we will work through in turn in this step.

### Recognizing that your struggles are understandable

It is really important to understand that the struggles you are having are part of a common human experience and relate to your history and your current ways of coping. To help you recognize that your struggles are understandable, you can reflect on what you know about our brains and bodies, your personal history, the situation you find yourself in and the ways in which you have learned to cope with difficult things. For example, you might continue your letter:

> *It is understandable that you would be worried about feeling depressed or anxious this week. In the past people often told you that you weren't capable or weren't good enough, and that is what your body has remembered. When you are struggling with difficult things, often these memories come to the surface, and you can remember when people put you down and criticized you when you tried to do new things. Of course, you would have learned from this that new things were too difficult to manage, or that your own feelings of inadequacy were the truth, rather than a feeling that was taught to you by other people. It is also understandable that your brain is very good at helping you make these feelings worse, by spending time ruminating and thinking about them, by pulling in other memories, or by thinking about new situations where things might be difficult, and focusing on how you might be rejected if you don't get things right. Your brain is also very good at helping you be sensitive to threats, particularly threats of being left alone or abandoned, because this is what all animals fear. In the past you found that food often helped you to deal with these painful feelings, or you ate with others to help you to fit in with people you thought would reject you.*

Sometimes, in fact quite often, we will find it hard to understand why we are struggling with things. For example, you may not recall your history in detail, or have a full understanding of why you cope in the way you do. When this happens it can be helpful to focus on what is threatening to you and what your biggest concerns would be if what you feel threatened by were actually to happen now. You can also look at the ways you have coped with these threats in the past. For example, what would worry you about stopping overeating or giving up dieting?

It is very likely that the threats you have experienced are those faced by all humans at some time in their lives, and your way of coping was the best you could find at the time. You may wish to discuss with someone close to you how you came to cope in these ways. If you don't want to, or there's no one suitable to talk to, it is important to recognize that your ways of coping have helped you, at least in the short term, so it is understandable that you would want to keep them until you had better ways of managing your feelings or difficult situations.

## Understanding the unintended consequences of the ways you have coped with threats

We do this not to beat ourselves up for doing things that in fact haven't solved difficulties for us, but to help us recognize some of the costs and pain that these ways of coping have caused us, and may cause us in the future. It is a part of recognizing our suffering and helps to motivate us to relieve it in a way that does not involve food. For example, our letter might continue:

> It is understandable that you would struggle with feelings of depression and anxiety. It is also understandable that the way you have learned to cope has been to withdraw, to hide away, not to want to share your feelings with anyone in case they hurt you or put you down, and to comfort eat. This way of coping with things has sometimes helped you get through difficult times in the past, but might stop you getting the support and care you need from people around you at the moment. It is also understandable that you bully yourself, to remind you to keep yourself safe from other people's

*attempts at attacking you. One of the unintended consequences is that you are now so good at bullying yourself that you end up feeling even more miserable, alone and isolated. It also stops you thinking about other ways of dealing with the things in your life that anybody would find difficult and challenging.*

## Understanding that it's *not* your fault but it *is* your responsibility

This is a key principle of compassion-focused therapy. Remember, we didn't ask to be born into the circumstances or relationships we grew up with, and we certainly did not ask to have a 'see-food-and-eat-it brain', a body that is better at storing food than burning it, and a complex emotional system that can easily get out of kilter! However, we have inherited these things and are responsible for managing them in a way that reduces our suffering and lets us take pleasure and joy in the life, body and brains that we have, and frees us to engage in the world around us.

So, to continue our letter, we might say:

*It's not your fault that you want to run away and hide – this is very normal for any of us when we are feeling under attack or under threat. Nor is it your fault that you didn't have an opportunity to learn that you are capable and can manage life's challenges. You didn't choose to be here, you didn't choose to have your history, you certainly didn't choose to have a brain that is primed for fear, or that is primed to ruminate on things you are finding difficult. You also didn't choose a brain that is set up to see food and eat it, or that responds so that food helps us with our feelings. Your overeating was encouraged when you grew up by other people, and the food industry, and it was the only way you could manage the painful feelings you had then and have now. Of course you overeat when you're socializing with other people – most people do – but for you this is a way of helping you get closer to other people so you don't feel so afraid that they will not want to be with you.*

*You do want to find other ways to cope with the threats you experience now, and I know you can and will work to find other ways to cope when you feel afraid that are better for you.*

## Step 7: Understanding what you need to help you cope with threats

The next step in letter writing focuses on understanding what you need to help you cope with your emotions or the situation you are in. This has two elements: what you needed in the past to help you find ways of coping, and what would help you to cope differently now.

### What did I need in the past?

For example, you might write:

> *In the past you needed people to support you, to mentor you, to help you feel confident in managing life's struggles, and to help you find ways of dealing with the challenges that all human beings face. This may have included people to tell you you were good at things, to teach you how to do things patiently, to tolerate your frustration when you couldn't cope any more, and to support you and help take over some of the things which you found too overwhelming. You may have needed people to be there for you when things were hard and to help remind you that you could deal with things as well. You also needed people not to use food to pacify your feelings.*

### What do I need to help me cope now?

What we have just written may well be very useful in helping us to identify our emotional and practical needs, but sadly we cannot change the past! However, knowing about these needs can help us to change the present and our future by responding to them in a different way. It can help put us in touch with the kinds of things we can say or do differently, rather than using our comfort food or dieting mind to get us through difficulties. So we might write:

> *The first thing you need to help you cope now is to recognize that you are facing difficult challenges at the moment – on top of the ones that every*

*human being faces, including dealing with your brain and body, you are also struggling with things at work that are difficult just now. You have too much work to do, and you are worried that people will judge you harshly if you can't do it all.*

*This is not unrealistic as there is an element of performance-related promotion in your job. However, what you need now are people to understand the amount of pressure that you are under, and to be supportive and sympathetic with that. You need to find ways to manage your workload differently, and perhaps to be more assertive with your managers. Try also to be honest with yourself about the things that make you good at your job, so that you don't feel so threatened when you are struggling with things. You may need to be able to share some of your worries with people at work who will be sympathetic and able to help you recognize that you are not the only one who's feeling under pressure at the moment.*

*You may need some structure and support to learn to deal with these difficult feelings and situations without using food. It may help to have a better structure to your eating, and to find other ways to deal with this stress so you are less likely to overeat. You may also need to accept that you will not be able to give up overeating all in one go, and to be gentle with yourself when you eat more than you need to.*

## Step 8: Developing compassionate coping thoughts and actions

The next part of your letter involves thinking about the ways of thinking and acting that may help you deal with the struggles you face in a different way. Remember that it is OK to allow yourself to keep your old ways of coping until you feel ready to give them up; otherwise this step can feel like making a list of things we *must* do, and we can then easily fall into the trap of beating ourselves up if we can't do them straight away or if some don't work for us. So in your compassionate letter you might say:

*Everybody struggles with work pressures, and you are no different from other people in that – remember how often in the past you have recognized that other people struggle at work and have tried to help them cope. Your friends and family may listen to your distress, and it is important that you listen to it too. In fact, several people have commented on the fact that you are overworking at the moment, and that you could slow down, and it would be OK. Perhaps you can look at what work you need to do and what you can schedule differently. Perhaps you can arrange a meeting with your manager to reschedule your workload.*

*You could also choose to eat with other people, as you know you are more likely to overeat at work when you are alone. Perhaps you could start by having lunch with Dave at work, so you are a little less hungry when you come home.*

Here we can see that a combination of thoughts and actions may be needed to help us cope differently.

It can help to write these thoughts and actions down in note form and keep them somewhere that's easy to get to when you want to remind yourself of them. People use various ways of doing this, for example jotting them down on a flashcard, or as a text or voice message on their phone. It can also help to remind ourselves of these thoughts and actions by saying them to ourselves via our compassionate image, or even in the mirror with a compassionate tone of voice.

It may well be that these new ways of coping do not feel at all comfortable, or even believable, at this point. That's absolutely normal. Part of the work you're doing in your letter is at least identifying that there are other ways of thinking about and managing threats that are different from the strategies you have learned in the past and used to help you cope.

## Step 9: Imagining a compassionate future

When you have developed some compassionate ways of thinking and acting differently to manage threats, it is important to think about how life would be if you could put these into practice. This will help you to explore compassionately the reasons why you might want to think and act differently in the future. One way to do this is to write about what your life would be like if you were able to follow the compassionate wisdom in your letter. So we focus on what could change and how things would be different. For example, you could write:

> *Kerry, I know it's really hard for you to think that you might deal with yourself in a more compassionate way around your mood, worries about work and comfort eating. However, if you were able to, perhaps you wouldn't feel so anxious and so fearful that other people are thinking critically of you. It might even be that you would feel under less stress at work. You might worry less about what you eat and be able to give up dieting. You might have a better balance between work and home life. You might even be able to enjoy your work more and take pleasure in your achievements there, and be content with the things you can achieve and tolerate the frustration of the things you can't.*

Clearly these are all 'maybes'; however, it is really important that this part of your letter helps you be open to these new ways thinking or acting. Just play around with them – write down all the possibilities you can think of.

It is likely that you will hear a lot of 'yes, buts' in your head when you are writing this part of your letter. Again, this is normal and to be expected; the key is to notice what the objections are but not to engage with them. If you feel that they are getting in the way, you can pause here in your letter and return to focusing on your compassionate image, feeling their concern for you and their real understanding of you, and knowing that they can help you with these concerns a little later in your letter. If need be, take a complete break from your letter at this point, and let your compassionate image help soothe the anxiety that thinking about new ways of being has prompted. When you feel ready, you can continue your letter.

## Step 10: Making a compassionate commitment to change

In this part of the letter your compassionate self will be supporting you and encouraging you to commit yourself to making some of the changes it suggested in Step 9. The key here is to commit to these changes without bullying yourself into making them. Your compassionate self is aware of your limitations, and so you can use it to help you decide what elements of compassionate thinking and action you are prepared to take on right now, and what may feel too difficult to try straight way. It is important to remember that you are moving towards these changes in a compassionate way, and that it is best to do this in small and achievable steps.

You may need at this point to re-read Step 9 from the perspective of your compassionate image ('you at your best' or your compassionate companion) to help identify the things that you feel you can move forward with now. Do remember that it takes courage to try new ways of coping, and wisdom to recognize what is possible for you in the short and then in the longer term. It can help to set out a series of steps that will take you gradually to the point where you can manage your distress in the ways your compassionate image would want you to.

So, for example, you might now write:

> *Kerry, having re-read my letter to you, I recognize that perhaps you are not as compassionate with yourself as you want to be, and a bit of you feels that this is your fault too! Perhaps you could try a couple of things to help you be more compassionate with yourself. Try not to blame yourself as much for the difficulties that you have faced at work, and let other people know that you are struggling and that maybe you need their support at this time.*

> *What you could try right now is to phone your best friend Mark, let him know you have had a hard week at work and plan to do something more relaxing together. You might talk to your boss, too, but you might need someone to help you do that. Maybe you could talk to Mark about how you could raise the idea with your boss that work has just got too difficult. You could also ask Dave to have lunch with you a couple of times in the week, and perhaps arrange for Danielle to visit you at the weekend, when you tend to be most likely to overeat when you feel down.*

> *You can practise bringing your compassionate image to mind to help you feel safer with your own feelings, and work on recognizing that they are not your fault.*

*I would like you to be compassionate with yourself all of the time, but we both know that this is impossible for any of us.*

*I know that you are going to find relaxing very difficult, as you normally feel driven to achieve things. But I would like you to try to do a self-soothing exercise for five minutes a day – though please don't be too hard on yourself if you find this difficult.*

Finally, think about how you can finish off your letter. You might do this by summarizing the main points of the letter, perhaps recognizing your courage for reading it, and wishing yourself well with the time to come.

For example, you might draw to a close by writing:

*Thank you for taking the time to read this, Kerry. You have faced some difficult decisions while you've been reading this letter, and explored some difficult feelings. This took a lot of courage on your part, and I am proud of you.*

*Good luck over the coming week. Please remember I will always be here for you if you need me.*

## Step 11: Paying compassionate attention to your letter

So now you've written your letter – to yourself. The final two steps are to do with you as the recipient as well as you as the writer.

Many people can write a very compassionate letter for someone else, or even for themselves, but cannot 'feel' it; these next two exercises are designed to help with this common difficulty.

### EXERCISE 14.1: IMAGINING OFFERING COMPASSION TO YOURSELF

The aim of this exercise is to help you 'feel' the compassion in your letter, to have the experience of being cared for and supported by another person in a warm, kind, non-judgemental and helpful way. This is similar to Exercise 5.13: again, you are going to imagine kindness and compassion flowing from you towards yourself.

When you feel ready, bring to mind your compassionate self. Imagine yourself expanding as if you are becoming calmer, wiser, stronger and more mature, and able to help.

Now imagine expanding the warmth within your body and imagine it flowing over and around you. Feel your genuine desire for you to be free of suffering and to flourish. Focus on your tone of voice. It can help to imagine having a conversation with yourself. Next think about your pleasure in being able to be kind to yourself and to accept your own kindness.

### Exercise 14.2: finding your compassionate voice

It is important to be able to 'hear' your letter in the voice you've used to write it. When we are being compassionate with others it is often the tone of our voice, far more than what we actually say, that conveys our compassion. In just the same way, it's not only what you say in your letter that is important, it's also the way you say it. So if you still find it difficult to feel and act on the compassion expressed in your letter, try this exercise, which involves reading your letter out loud to yourself.

Many people find it really helpful to read their letter out loud and listen to it carefully, as if they were being compassionate with somebody else. It can sometimes help to do this in front of a mirror, or to a photograph of yourself. If you tend to pick on yourself about size and shape, or how or what you eat, it may be better to look at just a picture of your face, rather than your whole body.

First, though, when you have written your letter, take time to pause and perhaps practise offering compassion to somebody else before you read it aloud to yourself. You might want to have a go at Exercise 5.7 in Chapter 5, focusing on finding your compassionate voice. Notice your tone of voice, the concern, the warmth, and the wisdom that your letter brings to somebody who is in pain and distress and just doing the best that they can to get through life, as we all are.

Now try reading your letter aloud to yourself. Sometimes it can be really helpful to record this and then listen to the recording from the perspective of yourself when you need compassion. This can make it a little easier to work out which parts of your letter are helpful to you. If you feel uncomfortable with this, just practise reading your letter aloud and notice which parts touch you and help you feel soothed and understood.

Often when we are feeling the need for compassion we are taken back to a place in our memory where we feel quite young, scared and unsupported. So you might find it helpful to read your letter to a younger version of yourself, as we tend naturally to be more compassionate towards children. Even so, many people who are highly self-critical can find this a struggle. Still – give it a go and see what helps you best to use the letter to offer compassion to yourself.

## Step 12: Enhancing your compassionate letter

As you read your letter to yourself, try to notice your feelings and whether they change as you read. Are there parts of your letter that are harsh or condemning? This is not at all unusual, particularly in the early stages of learning to be compassionate. If this is the case, you may wish to change these parts of your letter. However, as I said at the beginning of this sequence, it is important not to get caught up in trying to write the 'perfect letter': it only needs to be *good enough* to bring our soothing system into play and tone down our threat and drive systems enough to allow us to consider other ways of thinking or acting without getting caught up in old coping strategies. No letter you write is ever going to be perfect, no matter how much you practise – and believe me, I have had a fair amount of practice!

Re-reading the letter often helps you to see blocks to compassion and to pinpoint things you can't believe or find hard. It's important to be compassionate with these blocks and to recognize that they are a normal part of the process. You can use them to develop your letter further.

## Making time to write your letter

Letter writing can be a very time-consuming process while we are learning. As I said at the beginning of this chapter, you'll probably need to set aside about an hour at a time to practise. You may also find it difficult and frustrating at times. However, it is also empowering to discover that you have this ability and can improve it by practice. It's a skill like any other. We can all learn to play the piano – some of us find it harder than others, some of us take a lot more time than others to make progress, but it is something we can all become *good enough* at. The key message with compassionate letters is that they don't have to be perfect; they just have to be good enough to:

- help stimulate compassion for yourself, and help you to find other ways of feeling safe with your emotions, rather than being driven to do something about them instantly;

- develop new ways of thinking about yourself, and about your shared humanity;

- find new ways of coping that fit for you and that have fewer unintended consequences than your old ones that involved food and eating.

If your letters are getting in touch with painful feelings, writing them can be quite exhausting, and the feelings may stay around for a little while after you have finished. In this case it is important to practise compassionate behaviour towards yourself after you have stopped writing. Try to allow yourself at least half an hour afterwards when you are not doing stressful things. It can also help to have something soothing or distracting to do at this time. You might want to plan for this in advance using some of the techniques we explored in Chapter 6.

On the final page of this chapter I have included a summary of the key steps in compassionate letter writing.

## SUMMARY

This chapter has explored using letter writing as a way of helping you to use your compassionate mind to find new solutions to overeating. You may find that this tool helps you to make use of the practical steps to changing your eating outlined in this book.

Of course, many people do not like writing letters and the structured approach I have set out here can look a little daunting. Please don't be put off! Once you begin to write letters you may find that your letter naturally follows the flow I have outlined in this chapter. Indeed, this step-by-step process was developed by analysing actual letters people have written and seeing what was most helpful. The structure given here is only a suggestion, to provide you with some ways to stimulate your compassionate mind to help you. Indeed, many people have used the steps in the letter-writing sequence to help them in their compassion work without ever writing a single letter! For example, some people develop compassionate letters in their heads, but rather than writing them down they dictate to themselves, or write compassionate poems or songs – even draw compassionate cartoons! Whatever works for you is absolutely fine; remember, the key to compassion is knowing what is helpful in the moment.

In the next and final chapter we will briefly remind ourselves of the key points of a compassionate mind approach to beating overeating.

Before beginning your letter, get into a compassionate mindset by bringing your compassionate image into mind. Allow yourself at least half an hour to write your letter and plan something soothing or distracting to do when you have finished.

1  Begin by getting in touch with the feelings or situations you are likely to find difficult. Do this by imagining yourself being in the situation you are going to face. Jot them down quickly – don't stay here for long!

2  Step outside the feelings using mindfulness or your soothing breathing rhythm.

3  Activate feelings of safety by developing your safe place.

4  Bring to mind your compassionate image – your compassionate companion or 'you at your best'.

5  Begin your letter by recognizing your courage, your resilience and the ways you have coped, both recently and in the past.

6  Develop empathy and understanding for your difficulties:
   - They are understandable – be specific about your history and memories in previous ways of coping, and the key threats that you were trying to avoid.
   - Understand the unintended consequences of your current ways of managing these difficulties.
   - Remind yourself that these events and ways of coping are not your fault but they are your responsibility.

7  Consider what you need to help you cope with the difficulty.
   - What did I need in the past?
   - What do I need now?

8  Develop self-compassionate coping thoughts and behaviours to deal with the struggle differently.

9  Think about how your life would be different if you were able to be more self-compassionate.

10  Make a compassionate commitment to the changes you feel ready to make.

11  Pay compassionate attention to your letter:
   - Offer compassion to yourself.
   - Find your compassionate voice.
   - Re-read your letter out loud to yourself. Ideally, use an image of you, either in the mirror, or a recent or much earlier photo.

12  Listen with your heart and wisdom to anything that could help your letter become even more compassionate.

13  Plan to do something soothing or distracting when you finish your letter.

**Figure 14.1:** Steps for compassionate letter writing

# 15 A compassionate focus on eating: final thoughts

This final chapter will bring together some of the ideas that have run through the whole book. To begin with, here are ten key reminders:

(1) Our relationship with food and eating can be very complicated. We evolved with a 'see-food-and-eat-it' brain and body, and an emotional system to help us survive in a world full of threats. We did not evolve for a sedentary lifestyle in a world of plenty with a powerful food industry that has created a huge range of easily accessible and highly appetizing foods, many of which are high in fat and sugar. In a modern world where we are subject to far fewer direct physical threats but quite a lot of mental and emotional stress, our emotional systems can become very entangled with our eating.

(2) A desire to overeat, therefore, is *absolutely not your fault* but the result of a whole range of factors over many of which we have no control. So, no matter what you weigh or what you eat there's nothing to be ashamed about – no matter what society says: remember, in some societies plumpness is a sign of beauty and wealth! However, how you eat, and how you care for your body more generally, *is your responsibility* – and you can learn to eat and look after yourself in new ways that are better for your physical and emotional health than relying on overeating to cope.

(3) Learning to be compassionate – kindly and more relaxed about your eating, rather than anxious, depressed and self-critical – can be the first step on a journey towards these new ways of eating and taking responsibility for yourself.

(4) Learning why compassion is so beneficial for you, for example by understanding the 'three systems' model of our emotions, will help you to see the value of living more compassionately. Remember,

compassion is not about being soft or self-indulgent, or about letting our guard down. It's about developing a very important inner quality, related to how our brain works, that will help us face difficulties in our lives and cope with setbacks and disappointments.

(5) Learning to become more aware – more *mindful* – of the urges to eat and the act of eating, and then of the link between our emotions and our eating, is a key step. This book has given you many ideas for exploring how to become more aware of when, what and why you eat what you do. It will help you understand how eating might have come to have emotional significance for you, for example as a comfort eater.

(6) Understanding your personal history, in terms of how your eating styles have evolved over time, can be especially useful. You may want to explore these ideas again from time to time. Different things may occur to you at different points on your journey, and as you move on you may gain different insights into your personal history and its links to your overeating.

(7) Getting to understand your personal relationship with food can help you to develop new ways of dealing with food and your feelings – not in an aggressive, forcing way, but in a kind and compassionate way.

(8) Learning to stand back from setbacks, and being open, curious and kind about them, can help you understand what they were about, what triggered them, and how you might respond differently next time. Getting angry with yourself, or becoming depressed, when setbacks occur is only likely to lead to further episodes of overeating.

(9) Taking practical steps such as meal planning, choosing healthy eating, gradually switching from unhealthy foods to more healthy ones – for example, stopping buying foods you know tend to trigger overeating for you – will help to change your relationship with food. By these means you can gradually learn to trust your body's responses to eating, for example its natural signals of hunger and fullness, and allow yourself to enjoy eating again.

(10) Developing your compassionate mind, for example through imagery exercises, will strengthen your capacity for compassion, both towards

yourself and towards others. In working through this book you have learned how to develop your soothing system, to manage difficult emotional experiences and to tolerate and mindfully explore your feelings. The key principle underlying all these changes is the development of a compassionate mind approach to eating. In all kinds of situations from now on, you can practise asking yourself: What would compassionate attention be focused on here? What would compassionate thinking be in this situation? How can I behave compassionately to myself or others in these circumstances? If I take a breath and slow down and switch on my compassionate mind, how would it help me? Compassionate letter writing can be a great help in dealing with the challenges that lie ahead.

There are a lot of ideas in this book – you may even feel that there are too many, or that the prospect of change is too complex, difficult or over-whelming. The key is to go one step at a time. Try things out for yourself and see what you can use – if you only change one or two things, that's still helpful. Few of us follow manuals or recipes to the letter, if we're honest. But we also know that if we want to learn to drive, play a musical instrument or speak Spanish, the more we practise the better we'll get. If ever you have thought, 'This can't work for me,' wonder why you say that; treat your response as an interesting question rather than a definitive statement. Remember, your threat/protection system may be used to running your life! Try saying instead: 'Maybe this will work for me; let me give it a try.'

Don't be frightened of asking for help, either: there are increasing numbers of dietitians and organizations you can consult. Sometimes your family doctor can be very helpful in advising you on what is available locally. Many people find that having the support of others is really valuable – although keep in mind that diet groups that focus too much on weight loss, rather than healthy eating and healthy living, may not be such a good idea, particularly if you find that your 'dieting mindset' leads to overeating (and longer-term weight gain). None the less, sharing your thoughts and experiences with others, and feeling supported and understood by them, can be very helpful, and seeking support is a very compassionate thing to do. If you would like some guidelines on where you might look for support, try the 'Useful resources' section at the end of this book. If you prefer not to meet others in person, there are some options here for making contact on the internet or over the phone.

The 'Useful resources' section also contains information on where you can find help in becoming more self-compassionate, and in working on overeating. Take your time to explore the possibilities and use your compassionate wisdom to help you decide which ones are likely to be most helpful to you.

I hope that the compassionate mind approach set out in this book will help you learn to change unhelpful eating habits and enable you to enjoy the wonderful tastes, textures and smells of food, and the opportunity to share these with people you care about and who care for you.

All that remains for me to do is to send you many compassionate good wishes in your new and developing relationship with food and your body. As they say in compassionate practice:

> *May you be well.*
> *May you be happy.*
> *May you be free from suffering –*
> *And may you be compassionate with your eating!*

# Useful resources

## Books

### Compassion

Christopher Germer, *The Mindful Path to Self-Compassion: Freeing Your Self from Destructive Thoughts and Emotions*. New York: Guilford, 2009.

Jeffrey Hopkins, *Cultivating Compassion: A Buddhist Perspective*. New York: Doubleday, 2001.

Bikshu Sangharakshita, *Living with Kindness: The Buddha's Teaching on Metta*. London: Windhorse Publications, 2008.

If you're interested in a more evolutionary approach, have a look at the following:

Richard J. Davidson and Anne Harrington, eds, *Visions of Compassion: Western Scientists and Tibetan Buddhists Examine Human Nature*. New York: Oxford University Press, 2002.

Paul Gilbert, *Compassion: Conceptualisations, Research and Use in Psychotherapy*. London: Routledge, 2005.

Paul Gilbert, *The Compassionate Mind*. London: Constable Robinson, 2009; New York: New Harbinger, 2010.

Paul Gilbert, *Compassion Focused Therapy*. London: Routledge, 2010.

### Mindfulness

Jon Kabat-Zinn, *Coming to our Senses: Healing Ourselves and the World through Mindfulness*. New York: Piatkus, 2005.

Don Siegel, *The Mindful Brain*. New York: Norton, 2007.

Ronald Siegel, *The Mindful Solution*. New York: Guilford, 2010.

Thich Nhat Hanh, *The Miracle of Mindfulness*. London: Rider, 1991.

### Mindfulness and eating

Susan Albers, *Mindful Eating 101*. New York: Routledge, 2006.

## Eating and dieting

Linda Bacon, *Health at any Size*. Dallas: BenBella Books, 2008.

David Booth, *The Psychology of Nutrition*. London: Taylor & Francis, 1994.

Alexandra Logue, *The Psychology of Eating and Drinking*, 3rd edn. New York: Brunner-Routledge, 2004.

Gary Taubes, *The Diet Delusion*. London: Vermillion, 2008.

## The Dalai Lama

The Dalai Lama is the spiritual head of Buddhism, which can be seen as both a spiritual and a philosophical tradition. It is particularly valuable for its insights into human psychology, built up over thousands of years of meditation and introspective observation.

Dalai Lama, *The Power of Compassion*. London: Thorson, 1995.

Dalai Lama, ed. N. Vreeland, *An Open Heart: Practising Compassion in Everyday Life*. London: Hodder & Stoughton, 2001.

## The importance of affection in our lives

Louis Cozolino, *The Neuroscience of Human Relationships: Attachment and the Developing Brain*. New York: Norton, 2007.

Sue Gerhardt, *Why Love Matters: How Affection Shapes a Baby's Brain*. London: Brunner-Routledge, 2004.

# CDs for meditation

Two useful book/CD combinations are:

Jack Kornfield, *Meditation for Beginners*. New York: Bantam Books, 2004.

Dagsay Tulku Rinpoche, *The Practice of Tibetan Meditation: Exercises, Visualisations, and Mantras for Health and Well Being*. Rochester, VT: Inner Traditions, 2002. This book offers a very useful set of postures and exercises, along with a CD of mantras and instructions.

Some useful CDs that will guide you are:

Jeffrey Brantley, *Calming Your Anxious Mind: How Mindfulness and Compassion Can Free You from Anxiety, Fear and Panic*. New York: Harbinger, 2003.

Pema Chodron, *How to Meditate: A Practical Guide to Making Friends with your Mind*. Boulder, CO: Sounds True, 2007.

Paul Gilbert, *Overcoming Depression: Talks with Your Therapist*. London: Constable Robinson, 2008. Two CDs with a range of exercises, some of which (e.g. soothing rhythm breathing and compassionate images) are covered in this book.

Jon Kabat-Zinn, *Guided Mindfulness Meditation*. Boulder, CO: Sounds True, 2005.

Mark Williams, John Teasdale, Zindel Segal and Jon Kabat-Zinn, *The Mindful Way through Depression: Freeing Yourself from Chronic Unhappiness*. Boulder, CO: Sounds True, 2007.

# Websites

## Compassion

*Compassionate Mind Foundation (www.compassionatemind.co.uk)*

In 2007, Paul Gilbert and a number of colleagues (including myself) set up a charity called the Compassionate Mind Foundation. On this website, you'll find various essays and details of other sites that look at different aspects of compassion. You'll also find a lot of material that you can use for meditation on compassion, and links to many other related websites.

*Mind & Life Institute (www.mindandlife.org)*

The Dalai Lama has formed relationships with Western scientists to develop a more compassionate way of living. More information on this can be found on this website.

*Centre for Compassion and Altruism Research and Education (http://ccare.stanford.edu/)*

Website of an institution set up by Professor James Doty for international work for the advancement of compassion.

*Self-Compassion (www.self-compassion.org)*

This website is run by Dr Kristin Neff, one of the leading researchers into self-compassion.

## Eating disorders and overeating

*BEAT (www.b-eat.co.uk)*

Beat is the working name for the UK-based Eating Disorders Association. This charity offers a wide range of helpful information and support for people with eating disorders and disordered eating.

*Academy for Eating Disorders (AED) (www.aedweb.org)*

This is mainly a website for professionals working with people with eating disorders, but is also a good source of information for the public.

*National Eating Disorder Information Centre (www.nedic.ca)*

This is a Canadian non-profit organization founded in 1985 to provide information and resources on eating disorders and preoccupations with food and weight. One of its main goals is to inform the public about eating disorders and related issues. It also staffs a Canadian-based helpline.

*National Centre for Overcoming Overeating (www.overcomingovereating.com)*

A great resource for non-dieting approaches to eating, based in the USA.

*WIN the Rockies (http://www.uwyo.edu/WinTheRockies/default.html)*

This website is a helpful resource for individuals and communities who want to foster acceptance of all people irrespective of body size. It is based on the principles of body-size differences and size-acceptance, positive self-acceptance, physically active living and healthful and pleasurable eating.

*Nourishing Connections (http://www.nourishingconnections.com)*

The main focus of this organization is on giving up dieting. It has a lot of helpful articles and resources to help you get back in touch with your hunger and satiety system.

*Linda Bacon (http://www.lindabacon.org/resources.html)*

Linda has pioneered the Health At Every Size movement in the USA. This non-dieting approach to eating and health is becoming increasingly popular in the UK too. This website contains useful articles and downloads for individuals and healthcare providers.

# References

## Chapter 1: Understanding our relationship with food

*On maintenance of weight loss*: National Heart, Lung and Blood Institute Obesity Education and Innovation Expert Panel, 'Clinical guidelines on the identification, evaluation, and treatment of overweight and obesity in adults: the evidence report', *Obesity Research*, 6, 1998, 51S–209S.

## Chapter 2: Making sense of overeating, part 1: how our bodies work

*On blood sugar levels and appetite*: A. W. Logue, *The Psychology of Eating and Drinking*, 3rd edn (New York: Brunner-Routledge, 2004), p. 182.

*On the starve–eat cycle*: A. Keys, J. Broze and A. Henschel, *The Biology of Human Starvation*, Vol. 2 (Minneapolis: Minnesota University Press, 1950).

*On the body's natural tendency to increase physical activity to match increased energy intake*: J. A. Levine, N. L. Ebhardt and M. D. Jensen, 'Role of nonexercise activity thermogenesis in resistance to fat gain in humans', *Science*, 283, 1999, 212–14.

## Chapter 3: Making sense of overeating, part 2: eating and our feelings

*On how we learn to eat*: See D. A. Booth, *The Psychology of Nutrition* (London: Taylor & Francis, 1994). He provides a fascinating review of how we learn to eat, how our eating patterns change as we grow older, and the psychological and biological influences on eating.

*On emotional and hormonal fluctuations in adolescence*: http://en.wikipedia.org/wiki/Adolescence provides a good overview of this fascinating stage in our development and the challenges that it can present.

*On the threat system of emotional regulation*: R. F. Baumeister, E. Bratslavsky, C. Finkenauer and K. D. Vohs, 'Bad is stronger than good', *Review of General Psychology*, 5, 2001, 323–70.

*On the areas of our brain and hormones which respond to kindness*: See references in Paul Gilbert, *The Compassionate Mind* (London: Constable Robinson, 2009), ch. 5.

*On the psychological distress experienced by people coming to NHS weight loss services*: C. Webb, 'Psychological distress in clinical obesity: the role of eating disorder beliefs and behaviours, social comparison and shame', unpublished doctoral manuscript, University of Leicester, 2000.

## Chapter 10: Motivating yourself to change

*On psychological research on change*: J. W. Prochaska and C. C. DiClemente, 'Stages and processes of self-change of smoking: toward an integrative model of change', *Journal of Consulting and Clinical Psychology*, 51: 3, 1983, 390–5.

## Chapter 11: Working out what your body needs

*On sugar content in processed foods*: Information based on UK NHS guidelines for healthy eating. For more detailed advice on balanced healthy eating, see www.nhs.uk/Livewell/Goodfood/Pages/Healthyeating.aspxcomments

## Chapter 13: Towards a new way of eating: the final steps

*On establishing a sleep routine*: For more detailed help in managing sleep problems, see Colin Espie, *Overcoming Sleep and Insomnia Problems* (London: Constable Robinson, 2006).

# Extra worksheets

## Worksheet 1: Building your compassionate companion

| |
|---|
| How would you like your ideal caring, compassionate image to look/appear? What are its visual qualities? |
| How would you like your ideal caring, compassionate image to sound, e.g. tone of voice? |
| What other sensory qualities can you give to it, e.g. its smell or textures? |
| How would you like your ideal caring, compassionate image to relate to you? (For example: in a caring, warm, understanding way) |
| How would you like to relate to your ideal caring, compassionate image? (For example: allowing it to care for you, listening to its wisdom and concern for you) |

## Worksheet 1: Building your compassionate companion

| |
|---|
| How would you like your ideal caring, compassionate image to look/appear? What are its visual qualities? |
| How would you like your ideal caring, compassionate image to sound, e.g. tone of voice? |
| What other sensory qualities can you give to it, e.g. its smell or textures? |
| How would you like your ideal caring, compassionate image to relate to you? (For example: in a caring, warm, understanding way) |
| How would you like to relate to your ideal caring, compassionate image? (For example: allowing it to care for you, listening to its wisdom and concern for you) |

**Worksheet 2: Compassionate thought balancing**

| Overeating thoughts | Compassionate alternative thoughts |
| --- | --- |
| | |

**Worksheet 2: Compassionate thought balancing**

| Overeating thoughts | Compassionate alternative thoughts |
|---|---|
|  |  |

**Worksheet 3: My compassion practice diary**

| Day | Type of practice, time and how long for | Comments: what was helpful? |
|---|---|---|
| Monday | | |
| Tuesday | | |
| Wednesday | | |
| Thursday | | |
| Friday | | |
| Saturday | | |
| Sunday | | |
| Comments on week's practice | | |

*Source:* Reproduced with kind permission from the Compassionate Mind Foundation website.

**Worksheet 3: My compassion practice diary**

| Day | Type of practice, time and how long for | Comments: what was helpful? |
|---|---|---|
| Monday | | |
| Tuesday | | |
| Wednesday | | |
| Thursday | | |
| Friday | | |
| Saturday | | |
| Sunday | | |
| Comments on week's practice | | |

*Source:* Reproduced with kind permission from the Compassionate Mind Foundation website.

## Worksheet 4: My compassionate formulation for overeating

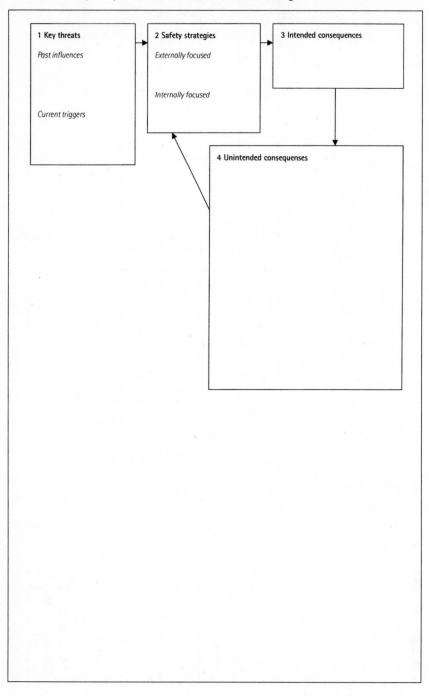

## Worksheet 4: My compassionate formulation for overeating

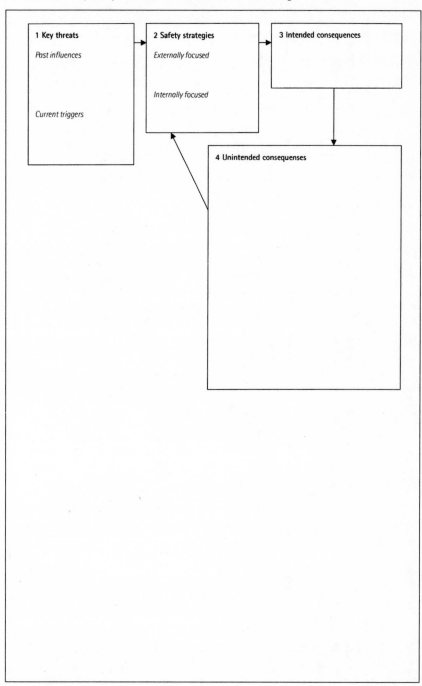

**Worksheet 5: Your eating diary**

Monday 23 March

| Situation<br>Where were you?<br>Who were you with?<br>How were you feeling?<br>What were you thinking before you ate? | What you ate or drank (type and amount)<br><br>Physical activity (type and duration) | Overeating?<br>Yes/No | Dieting mindset or comfort food mindset active when eating?<br>Yes/No | Thoughts and feelings<br>These can be thoughts and feelings during or after eating, about doing the diary, or anything else that you think is important |
|---|---|---|---|---|
| | | | | |

**Worksheet 5: Your eating diary**

| Monday 23 March | | | |
| --- | --- | --- | --- |
| Situation<br>Where were you?<br>Who were you with?<br>How were you feeling?<br>What were you thinking before you ate? | What you ate or drank (type and amount)<br>Physical activity (type and duration) | Overeating?<br>Yes/No | Dieting mindset or comfort food mindset active when eating?<br>Yes/No | Thoughts and feelings<br>These can be thoughts and feelings during or after eating, about doing the diary, or anything else that you think is important |
| | | | | |

**Worksheet 6: Managing blocks to monitoring**

| My personal blocks | Compassionate things I can say to myself or do to get past the block |
| --- | --- |
| | |

**Worksheet 6: Managing blocks to monitoring**

| My personal blocks | Compassionate things I can say to myself or do to get past the block |
|---|---|
|  |  |

**Worksheet 7: Diary review sheet**

Eating pattern
How long do I leave between eating episodes?                    _____ hours
How many times per day do I eat more often than every 3–4
hours?                                                          _____
How many times do I eat less often than every 3–4 hours?       _____

Energy needs
What is my daily energy need?                                  _____ calories
How much energy do I take in each day?                         _____ calories
How much energy do I use up each day?                          _____ calories
Am I eating more or less than I need each day?                 More/Less

What I eat and drink
Are there specific types of food that trigger overeating?

Are there any foods that help me not to overeat?

Are there any things I take into my body that affect my appetite (e.g. medication,
drugs, alcohol)?

Times, people, places
Are there any times, people or places that make overeating more likely?

Are there any times, people or places that protect me from overeating?

My feelings and overeating
Are there any feelings that make my overeating worse?

Are these physical sensations, such as hunger?

Are these emotions, such as sadness, boredom, anger, anxiety?

My thoughts and overeating
Am I in a dieting mindset before, during or after overeating?            Yes/No
Am I in a comfort food mindset before, during or after overeating?       Yes/No
Do I give myself permission to overeat as a treat?                       Yes/No
Do I use overeating to punish myself?                                    Yes/No
Do I hope that overeating will help me manage difficult feelings, memories,
or events?                                                               Yes/No
Do I follow certain rules or habits that I have been taught about eating?  Yes/No
Do I criticize or bully myself about what I have eaten or the way that I eat?  Yes/No
Am I worried about what other people will think about my overeating?     Yes/No

*If you answer 'yes' to any of these questions, try to be as specific as you can about
exactly what you are thinking and, if you can, where you learned to think in this way.*

**Worksheet 7: Diary review sheet**

Eating pattern
How long do I leave between eating episodes?                    _____ hours
How many times per day do I eat more often than every 3–4
hours?                                                                          _____
How many times do I eat less often than every 3–4 hours?   _____

Energy needs
What is my daily energy need?                                        _____ calories
How much energy do I take in each day?                          _____ calories
How much energy do I use up each day?                          _____ calories
Am I eating more or less than I need each day?               More/Less

What I eat and drink
Are there specific types of food that trigger overeating?

Are there any foods that help me not to overeat?

Are there any things I take into my body that affect my appetite (e.g. medication,
drugs, alcohol)?

Times, people, places
Are there any times, people or places that make overeating more likely?

Are there any times, people or places that protect me from overeating?

My feelings and overeating
Are there any feelings that make my overeating worse?

Are these physical sensations, such as hunger?

Are these emotions, such as sadness, boredom, anger, anxiety?

My thoughts and overeating
Am I in a dieting mindset before, during or after overeating?          Yes/No
Am I in a comfort food mindset before, during or after overeating?  Yes/No
Do I give myself permission to overeat as a treat?                         Yes/No
Do I use overeating to punish myself?                                          Yes/No
Do I hope that overeating will help me manage difficult feelings, memories,
or events?                                                                            Yes/No
Do I follow certain rules or habits that I have been taught about eating?  Yes/No
Do I criticize or bully myself about what I have eaten or the way that I eat?  Yes/No
Am I worried about what other people will think about my overeating?  Yes/No

*If you answer 'yes' to any of these questions, try to be as specific as you can about
exactly what you are thinking and, if you can, where you learned to think in this way.*

**Worksheet 8: Nine key questions for analysing the relationship between eating and the three emotional systems**

1   Am I at greater risk of overeating when my threat/protection system comes into play?

2   What types of threat are most likely to trigger my overeating?

3   Are there any other threats that I pay attention to once my threat/protection mindset is active?

4   How does eating help me to cope when my threat/protection system is switched on?

5   Does eating help me to feel soothed?

6   Does eating help me turn off or tone down the threat/protection system?

7   Does eating activate my drive/achievement system?

8   How do I hope that eating will make me feel safer?

9   What are the unintended consequences of overeating?

**Worksheet 8: Nine key questions for analysing the relationship between eating and the three emotional systems**

1   Am I at greater risk of overeating when my threat/protection system comes into play?

2   What types of threat are most likely to trigger my overeating?

3   Are there any other threats that I pay attention to once my threat/protection mindset is active?

4   How does eating help me to cope when my threat/protection system is switched on?

5   Does eating help me to feel soothed?

6   Does eating help me turn off or tone down the threat/protection system?

7   Does eating activate my drive/achievement system?

8   How do I hope that eating will make me feel safer?

9   What are the unintended consequences of overeating?

**Worksheet 9: My new compassionate formulation for overeating**

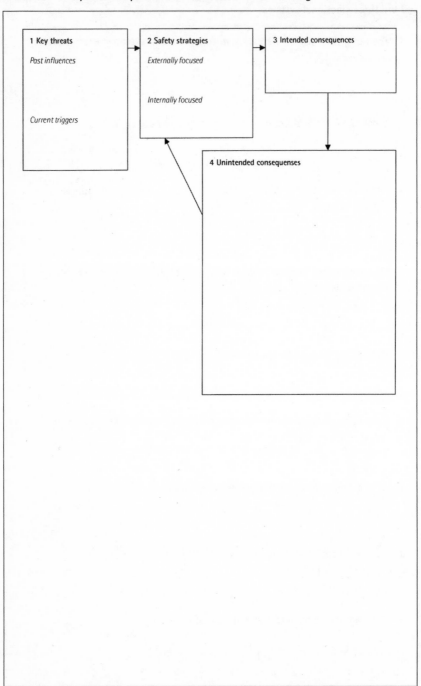

## Worksheet 9: My new compassionate formulation for overeating

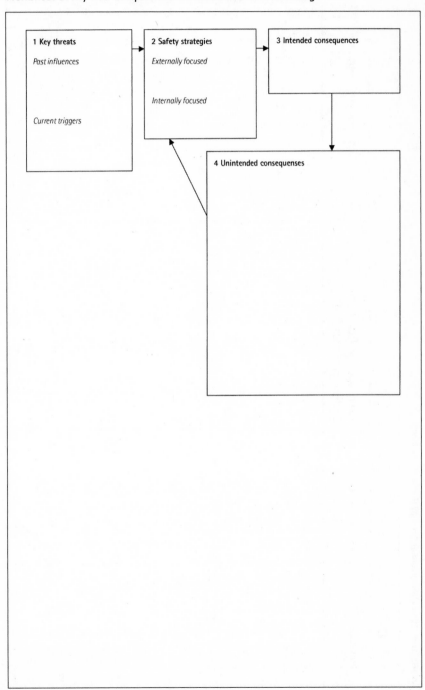

**1 Key threats**

*Past influences*

*Current triggers*

**2 Safety strategies**

*Externally focused*

*Internally focused*

**3 Intended consequences**

**4 Unintended consequenses**

Worksheet 10a: Daily food intake and energy balance

(a) Daily record

| Food eaten | Approximate energy intake (calories) | Main food type (starch, fruit/veg., protein, dairy, sugar/fat) | Activity and approximate energy used |
|---|---|---|---|
| | | | |

Worksheet 10b: Daily food intake and energy balance

(b) Daily and weekly summary

| | Monday | Tuesday | Wednesday | Thursday | Friday | Saturday | Sunday | Weekly summary |
|---|---|---|---|---|---|---|---|---|
| Total calorie intake | | | | | | | | |
| Starch | | | | | | | | |
| Fruit and vegetables | | | | | | | | |
| Protein | | | | | | | | |
| Dairy | | | | | | | | |
| Sugar and fat | | | | | | | | |
| Alcohol | | | | | | | | |
| Energy need ( = 2,000 for female/ 2,500 for male + extra for energy expended in activity) | | | | | | | | |
| Energy balance ( = calorie intake − energy need) | | | | | | | | |

Worksheet 10a: Daily food intake and energy balance

(a) Daily record

| Food eaten | Approximate energy intake (calories) | Main food type (starch, fruit/veg., protein, dairy, sugar/fat) | Activity and approximate energy used |
|---|---|---|---|
| | | | |

Worksheet 10b: Daily food intake and energy balance

(b) Daily and weekly summary

| | Monday | Tuesday | Wednesday | Thursday | Friday | Saturday | Sunday | Weekly summary |
|---|---|---|---|---|---|---|---|---|
| Total calorie intake | | | | | | | | |
| Starch | | | | | | | | |
| Fruit and vegetables | | | | | | | | |
| Protein | | | | | | | | |
| Dairy | | | | | | | | |
| Sugar and fat | | | | | | | | |
| Alcohol | | | | | | | | |
| Energy need (=2,000 for female/ 2,500 for male + extra for energy expended in activity) | | | | | | | | |
| Energy balance (=calorie intake − energy need) | | | | | | | | |

**Worksheet 11: Daily meal plan sheet**

| Meal or snack | Time and place | Food and drink to be taken | Comments, including any problems in keeping to meal plan, any solutions to these problems or changes to the plan |
|---|---|---|---|
| Breakfast | | | |
| Mid-morning snack | | | |
| Lunch | | | |
| Mid-afternoon snack | | | |
| Evening meal | | | |
| Evening snack | | | |
| Supper | | | |

**Worksheet 11: Daily meal plan sheet**

| Meal or snack | Time and place | Food and drink to be taken | Comments, including any problems in keeping to meal plan, any solutions to these problems or changes to the plan |
|---|---|---|---|
| Breakfast | | | |
| Mid-morning snack | | | |
| Lunch | | | |
| Mid-afternoon snack | | | |
| Evening meal | | | |
| Evening snack | | | |
| Supper | | | |

**Worksheet 12: Managing blocks to regular eating**

| Practical or emotional block to managing regular eating | Compassionate things I can say to myself or do to get past the block |
|---|---|
| | |
| | |
| | |
| | |
| | |
| | |

**Worksheet 12: Managing blocks to regular eating**

| Practical or emotional block to managing regular eating | Compassionate things I can say to myself or do to get past the block |
|---|---|
|  |  |
|  |  |
|  |  |
|  |  |
|  |  |
|  |  |

**Worksheet 13: High-risk foods for overeating**

| Food | Comfort food? Yes/No | Enjoyable food? Yes/No | Treat food? Yes/No | Self-punishing food? Yes/No |
|------|------|------|------|------|
|      |      |      |      |      |
|      |      |      |      |      |
|      |      |      |      |      |
|      |      |      |      |      |
|      |      |      |      |      |
|      |      |      |      |      |
|      |      |      |      |      |
|      |      |      |      |      |
|      |      |      |      |      |
|      |      |      |      |      |
|      |      |      |      |      |
|      |      |      |      |      |
|      |      |      |      |      |
|      |      |      |      |      |
|      |      |      |      |      |
|      |      |      |      |      |
|      |      |      |      |      |
|      |      |      |      |      |
|      |      |      |      |      |
|      |      |      |      |      |

**Worksheet 13: High-risk foods for overeating**

| Food | Comfort food? Yes/No | Enjoyable food? Yes/No | Treat food? Yes/No | Self-punishing food? Yes/No |
|------|------|------|------|------|
|  |  |  |  |  |
|  |  |  |  |  |
|  |  |  |  |  |
|  |  |  |  |  |
|  |  |  |  |  |
|  |  |  |  |  |
|  |  |  |  |  |
|  |  |  |  |  |
|  |  |  |  |  |
|  |  |  |  |  |
|  |  |  |  |  |
|  |  |  |  |  |
|  |  |  |  |  |
|  |  |  |  |  |
|  |  |  |  |  |
|  |  |  |  |  |
|  |  |  |  |  |
|  |  |  |  |  |
|  |  |  |  |  |

**Worksheet 14: Dealing with blocks to meal planning**

| Practical and emotional blocks to managing a meal plan | Compassionate things I can say to myself or do to help me manage my meal plan |
|---|---|
| | |
| | |
| | |
| | |
| | |
| | |
| | |

**Worksheet 14: Dealing with blocks to meal planning**

| Practical and emotional blocks to managing a meal plan | Compassionate things I can say to myself or do to help me manage my meal plan |
| --- | --- |
| | |
| | |
| | |
| | |
| | |
| | |
| | |

**Worksheet 15: Tomorrow's meal plan**

| Day and date | | |
|---|---|---|
| Eating episode | Time | Food and drink to be taken (including type and amount) |
| Breakfast | a.m. | |
| Mid-morning snack | a.m. | |
| Lunch | p.m. | |
| Mid-afternoon snack | p.m. | |

| Evening meal | p.m. | | Supper | p.m. | |
|---|---|---|---|---|---|
| | | | | | |

**Worksheet 15: Tomorrow's meal plan**

| Day and date | | |
|---|---|---|
| Eating episode | Time | Food and drink to be taken (including type and amount) |
| Breakfast | a.m. | |
| Mid-morning snack | a.m. | |
| Lunch | p.m. | |
| Mid-afternoon snack | p.m. | |

| Evening meal | p.m. | | Supper | p.m. | |
|---|---|---|---|---|---|
| | | | | | |

# Index

Index note: entries of particular importance appear in bold type. Entries for charts, worksheets and tables appear in italics.

adolescence   52–3
advertising   7–8, 10, 22, 62
alcohol   35, 36–7, 61, 62, 296
anorexia   6, 18

binge eating   6, 13, 43, 44–5
**blocks (managing)**
  about changing eating patterns   227–30, 232, 264–5, *265, 266*
  about food monitoring   189, 192, *193*, 194, *194*, 195
  about meal planning   275–6, *277, 278*
  about self-compassion   152, 156–62, 295
blood sugar   20, 42, 238, 239, 240
  *see also* energy balance
BMI (Body Mass Index)   18, 28, *29–30*
body types   20–2, 27–8
breathing techniques   99–101
Buddhism   68–9, 96, 113
bulimia   6, 18, 43

caffeine   35–6, 296
calorie regulation   46–7, 74, 197, 236, 239–40, 241–3, 246–8, 251, *252–3*, 254, 279
  *see also* **changing eating patterns**; nutritional needs
carbohydrates   237, *238, 239*
**changing eating patterns**   225, 257–8, 320
  action and maintenance   221, 223
  changing food associations   290–2
  dealing with blocks and setbacks   227–30, 232, 264–5, *265, 266*
  dealing with trigger foods   267, *268–9*, 270–2, 273

lapse and termination stages   221–2
pre-contemplation and contemplation stages   220, 223
preparation stage   220–1, 223, 226, 227
process of change   219–23, 233
regulating meal times   258–60, *261–2*, 263–4, 273
using compassionate motivation   223–7, 232
  *see also* compassionate mind development; **diaries**; letter writing (compassionate); meal planning; nutritional needs; **overeating (influences)**
childhood and children   4, 5, 25, 28, 51–2, 58, 62–3, 77, 165
  *see also* overeating (influences)
comfort eating   4–6, 26, 51, 55, 58–60, 77–9, 131–2, *132*, 267
  *see also* **changing eating patterns**; compassionate mind development; overeating (influences); soothing systems
**compassionate mind development**   1–2, 9–10, 82–3, 93–4, **105–14**, 129–30
  compassion and care for well-being   87–8
  compassion towards others   114–18
  compassion towards overeating   114–15, 117–18
  compassion towards self   118–20, 125–9
  compassionate attention/ concentration   83, 95–7, 98–9, 101–2
  compassionate behaviour   84, 150–2
  compassionate emotions and motives   84–5

compassionate empathy and
non-judgment  90–1
compassionate imagery  85, 94–5
*see also* **exercises**
compassionate motivation  85, 223–7, 232
compassionate sensitivity and
sympathy  88–9
compassionate thinking and
reasoning  84, 144–5, *145*, 146, *147*,
148–50
distress tolerance  89–90
**exercises**  98–101, 103–4, 110–14, 115–18,
119–20, 121–3, 126–9, 142–3, 144–5,
159–61, 176, 225–7, 231, 242, 255–6,
259–60, 264–5, 275–6, 288–9, 291, 292
*see also* **letter writing (compassionate)**
Gilbert's compassion circle  *87*, 87–92
mental blocks about  152, 156–62, 295
nature of compassion  68–70
safe places  102–5, 139, 176, 247, 302
self-correction  148–50, *149*
stress toleration  141–3
using developed skills  223–5, 242, 255–6,
259, 276, 287, 291, 292, 300–18
your compassionate companion  120–5,
*124*, 126–8, 139, 142, 176, 224, 300–1
*see also* **blocks (managing); changing
eating patterns; diaries;** diets; emotions;
**imagery and compassion; letter writing
(compassionate); mindsets; overeating
(influences);** self-criticism; **soothing
system;** Western society
culture *see* Western society

dairy and milk products  237, *238*, *239*, 296
depression  1, 9, 10, 18, 39–40, 63
*see also* **compassionate mind development;**
drive/achievement systems; mindsets
(dieting); **self-criticism;** soothing
systems; threat/protection systems
diabetes  10–11

diaries  225, 227, 288
blocks about keeping  189, 192, *193*, 194,
*194*, 195
developing compassionate self  152, *153*,
*154–5*
eating patterns  184, *185*, 186–9, *190–1*, 194,
243, *244*, 254, 259–60, 265, 267, *268*, 287
reviewing  195–9, *200*, 201–2
*see also* **changing eating patterns;** letter
writing (compassionate); record keeping
and list making
diets  10–13, 25–6, 28–9, 31–2, 39, 56–7, 60,
172–3
chaotic eating  43–5
effect of rules  63–7
mindset  70, 73–7, *76*, 78–9, 82, 144, 205, 294
starve-binge-purge cycle  42–3, *44*, 48
starve-eat cycle  37–42, 48
*see also* **changing eating patterns;** comfort
eating; **compassionate mind
development;** drive/achievement
systems; **meal planning; nutritional
needs; overeating (influences);** physical
activity
digestion  46
disorders *see* eating disorders
distraction techniques  138–41
drinking  33–5, 36–7, 286
**drive/achievement system**  53, *54*, 56–7, 60,
75–7, 133, 205, 207, 209, 211, 301
*see also* diets; mindsets; socializing
drugs  35–6

eating disorders  6, 18, 43, 44
eating patterns  37–45, *44*, 48, 51–2
*see also* **changing eating patterns; comfort
eating; compassionate mind
development; diaries;** diets;
**drive/achievement systems; evolution;
mindsets; overeating (influences);
threat/protection systems**

emotions   1, 5–7, 9–10, 13, 14, 15–18, 28–9, 50–1, *54*, 60–7
   *see also* **comfort eating; compassionate mind development; drive/achievement systems; letter writing (compassionate); mindsets; soothing systems; threat/protection systems**
energy balance   45–9, 196–7, 234, 236, 248, *249*, *250*, 251, *252–3*, *254–5*, 270
evolution   1–5, 7, 19–20, 31, 84, 86
exercise *see* physical activity
**exercises** (for compassionate mind development)   98–101, 103–4, 110–14, 115–18, 119–20, 121–3, 126–9, 142–3, 144–5, 159–61, 176, 225–7, 231, 242, 255–6, 259–60, 264–5, 275–6, 288–9, 291, 292
   *see also* **letter writing (compassionate); soothing systems**

family and friends *see* socializing; support
famine *see* evolution; starvation diets
fashion   21–3
fats and sugars   237–8, *238*, *239*
food *see* **changing eating patterns**; comfort eating; compassionate mind development; diets; meal planning; nutritional needs; overeating (influences)
food industry   7–8, 11, 28, 62, 132
fruit and vegetables   3, 19, 237, *238*, *239*, 281
fullness (responding to)   281, 286–9

glycogen   34–5
guilt *see* self–criticism

health   23–4, 28, 29–31, 293–5
help *see* support
hunger   21, 32, 33, 42–3, 44–5, 281, 286–90

imagery and compassion   85, 94–5
   distractions techniques   139–40
   safe places   102–5, 139, 176, 247, 302
   stress toleration   142–3
   *see also* **compassionate mind development; exercises (for compassionate mind development)**
insulin   20, 35

laxatives   35–6
**letter writing (compassionate)**   160, 227, 232, 291, 315–17
   getting started   299–300
   quick guide to   301–315, 318
   *see also* **compassionate mind development; soothing systems**

**meal planning**   279–80, *282–5*, 320
   benefits   274–5
   dealing with problems   275–6, 277, *278*
   nutritional balance   280–1
   responses to hunger and fullness   281, 286–90
   *see also* **changing eating patterns; diaries; nutritional needs**
meat and fish   3, 237, *238*, *239*
media   11–12, 23, 61, 140, 296
mental blocks *see* blocks (managing)
metabolism   20–1, 32, 40, 42, 45–7
   *see also* nutritional needs; set-point system
milk *see* dairy products
mindfulness   69, 96–7, 98–101, 102, 139, 272, 286–9, 320
   *see also* **compassionate mind development**; mindsets; soothing systems
**mindsets**   79–81, 106–7, 146, 148, 188
   developing compassionate   70, *70*, 73, 81, 82–3, 93–4, **105–30**, 176, 223–5
   dieting   *70*, 73–7, *76*, 78–9, 82, 144, 205, 294